Vibrant Health Now!

How to use essential oils, aromatherapy and
natural health products to detox your body
and reach optimal health

Casey Conrad & Alan Simpson

www.KeysToYoungLiving.com

Published by:
Communication Consultants WBS, Inc.
11 Kenyon Avenue
Wakefield, RI 02879
401-792-7009

Disclaimer:
The information contained herein is for educational purposes only and as a guideline for personal use. It should not be used as a substitute for medical counseling with a health professional. Neither the authors nor the publisher accepts responsibility for such use.

Table of Contents

Introduction

I firmly believe that everything happens for a reason, and yet my introduction into the world of essential oils would seem a complete fluke. It all began when I was a speaker at a health and fitness convention in Sydney, Australia. Between the two speaking sessions I was giving that day I had some time to kill and roamed into the trade show area. I found myself in the wellness section and came upon a single booth that caught the attention of my olfactory senses.

A man stood at the counter speaking to a captivated group of people. What he was doing made me laugh; he had a bottle of Peppermint essential oil in his hand above his head and was letting drops of it fall into his mouth. He then proceeded to put some of the oil into his hand, rub it all over his face and let out an exhilarating "ahhhhh." He then said something like, "You would never be able to do that with the Peppermint oil you buy at a health food store." While laughing I thought to myself, "this guy is a nut," but his energy level, enthusiasm, and group of wide-eyed listeners made me pause to hear more.

He began rattling off a list of maladies that Peppermint oil could help: Digestion, congestion, upset stomach, low energy, and pain were just a few. Being the daughter of a surgeon, I grew up running around an emergency room and using pharmaceuticals without question; I initially snickered at such a laundry list of applications that one simple little bottle of Peppermint could aid. But, as chance would have it this guy said the magic word that just so happened to resonate with me in that moment—pain.

Three months prior to my arriving in Sydney, I had found myself one morning in such excruciating back pain that I was unable to get out of bed. This was particularly strange and shocking because I have been an athlete all my life and am in great shape. Aside from a small amount of discomfort in my back the day before—which had become the "norm" after intense exercise or excessive yard work—I had no warning that this total incapacitation was about to happen.

The good part about being from a doctor's family is the ease at which you can get assistance, and it just so happened that the father of one of my business partners is an osteopath. With one call I was able to get the drugs that allowed me temporary relief to gingerly get out of bed, get some clothes on (with assistance) and be driven to his office for a spinal adjustment.

I was a mess for almost two weeks. It took several minutes to get out of bed each morning. I couldn't bend over, and needed help to even put on my shoes! I would start to feel a little bit better but then have a setback if I did any type of exercise or even light gardening. It was frustrating and to me inconceivable—especially since I had been doing yoga for six years and hadn't done any high impact exercise for over a decade.

This went on for a couple of months until my father suggested that I go see an orthopedic surgeon to try and get some answers. After one visit, the doctor suggested an MRI since nothing was obvious from an examination and x-ray. $1,000 + later in expenses not covered by my wonderful insurance company the answer was grim; "your L-1 and L-2 are compressed due to the abuse you gave your body over the years. There is nothing you can do about it except manage it and hope it doesn't get bad enough to need surgery."

Surgeon's kid or not, I am not a fan of anything that involves cutting my body, and I wasn't at all happy with "there's nothing you can do." So I began to do research on the Internet about back health. I invested in books, DVD's and other back-strengthening programs. I religiously did specific exercises daily and had enough improvement that I could at least exercise enough to feel better emotionally. I began to gain some strength back and be well enough for the trip to Sydney but the reality was that I was only managing the back pain and needed to take a lot of ibuprofen daily.

So when this seemingly crazy guy mentioned Peppermint could help with muscle pain, I stepped up and asked the question, "How does an oil act as a pain reliever?" Well, you would think I opened the Encyclopedia Britannica! He went off into this very technical explanation about the medicinal properties in Peppermint and several other oils that quickly reminded me of why I nearly failed out of Chemistry in high school.

Fortunately he must have seen the glossed over look in my eyes and in an effort to gain back my interest said, "Do you have some pain?" I simply said, "Yes, my lower back." Without asking me any other questions he offered to put some oils on my back so I could see for myself whether or not they gave me relief. After 24 hours of sitting in a plane only two days earlier, I was willing to give anything a try. Besides, I'm adventurous.

He pulled me into the booth, had me take off my blazer and bend over a chair. He un-tucked and pushed my shirt halfway up my back and began to put drops of several different oils up and down my spine, feathering them in with a light, sweeping motion of his fingers. I don't even know how many different oils he put on but I could see at least six or seven. I was due to speak again in 30 minutes, so I thanked him and left the booth without getting to ask all my questions.

To reach the auditorium that I was speaking in, it was about a ten-minute walk. Around three minutes into the trip I began to realize that my back wasn't hurting as much as it had been prior to the application of oils. I must admit I thought to myself, "Is that possible? Could my back really be hurting less because this nutty guy put a bunch of oils on it?" It wasn't until I finished my 90-minute lecture that I really had the time to stop and realize that I hadn't had any back pain while speaking. Amazing!

Introduction

I immediately made my way back into the trade show area before it closed for the day. I located the booth and was excited to see that the nutty guy was still there. He recognized me and asked, "How's your back feeling?" I replied, "Okay, you got me; what the heck did you put on my back?" It was his turn to laugh and he replied, "I used the oils to perform the Raindrop Technique." My only reply was, "I want to buy them right now. I don't care what they cost." Although I was crushed when he told me "I don't sell them and only have my own supply here with me," I was happy to learn where I could get these oils before I left the country.

That nutty guy was Alan Simpson the co-author of this book. Never in my wildest dreams could I have ever predicted that my chance meeting of him and his wife Linda would have such a huge impact on my life both personally and professionally. Since that fateful day I have become a prolific user and advocate of essential oils and have spoken to people around the world about oils and oil-enhanced products. Now I am publishing this book.

I'm not sure how you got this book or why you have been introduced to essential oils, but I'm glad for it. My only hope is that by incorporating essential oils into your life and by making better nutritional and personal care choices, you will enjoy the same number of benefits that I have.

In good health,

Casey Conrad

Setting the Stage

Author's note:

You're interested in vibrant health and yet the first section of this book is filled with information and statistics on the sad state of health in Western society. Why? Because understanding the history of disease states sets the stage for a greater appreciation of the lifestyle changes we suggest throughout this book. However, we recognize that not everyone enjoys statistics—especially gloomy ones! Therefore, we did not make this information a chapter but rather a section entitled "Setting the stage." We hope that you take the time to read it, or at least skim through it.

Vibrant Health Now! Everyone wants to be vibrant and healthy and most want it now. Think about this: The top 5 categories in the global wellness industry generate over <u>one trillion dollars</u> (US$) in annual revenue[1]. The categories are 1) Beauty and Anti-Aging with $679 billion, 2) Fitness & Mind-Body Exercise with $390 billion, 3) Healthy

---

[1] www.statista.com/statistics/168576/market-size-of-the-wellness-industry-by-segment/

Eating/Nutrition & Weight Loss with $276 billion, 4) Preventative/Personalized Health with $243 billion, and 5) Complimentary & Alternative Medicine with $113 billion.

According to BCC Research Market Forecasting, the global anti-aging market for just the Baby Boomer generation is enjoying a compounded annual growth rate of over 11%.[2] The reason that all these segments continue to grow, even through difficult economic times, is because the desire to look young and feel healthy is resilient in even the worst of financial times.

Let's face it, whether it is the latest machine or exercise for flatter abs or greater muscle tone; a facial product for fewer lines, wrinkles or age spots; a nutritional supplement for more energy or less aches and pains, or perhaps a diet to lose some weight, Western society has a love affair with looking good and feeling younger.

In some respects we've done a pretty good job, at least in the aesthetics' area. Gone are the days when you received Geritol on your 40th birthday or succumbed to blue-grey hair by the time you were 50. 60 isn't just the new 50—it's the new 40! Botox treatments, Pilate's classes, a private personal trainer and regular visits to hair salons and spa's have all empowered people to look younger.

Further, if you looked only at the actuarial tables for Western cultures, the statistics show that we aren't just obsessed with anti-aging, we are achieving longer life

---

[2] http://www.bccresearch.com/report/anti-aging-products-services-hlc060a.html

spans. In 1900, the average life expectancy for Americans was 48 for men and 51 for women. In 1960, the average was 67 and 74, respectively, and in 2005 it was 75 and 81.[3] When you consider how many years man has inhabited the world, this is an incredible feat; we have increased life expectancy by an average of almost 60% in just 105 years.

What does longer get us?

Although modern science and medicine have allowed us to increase our lifespan, are we actually living more vibrant, healthy lives? In that same 105-year span, the number of diseases and debilitating conditions present in western societies has exploded. Chronic diseases such as heart disease, stroke, cancer, diabetes, and arthritis are the leading causes of death and disability in the US, accounting for 7 out of every 10 deaths. According to the Center for Disease Control, (CDC), 133 million Americans—almost 1 out of every 2 adults—has at least one chronic illness.

Cancer. Cancer in the United States has escalated to pandemic proportions. According to the National Cancer

---

According to the Center for Disease Control, (CDC), 133 million Americans—almost 1 out of every 2 adults—has at least one chronic illness.

---

[3] National Vital Statistics Report, Vol. 59, No. 9, September 28, 2011

Institute, 1,596,670 men and women will be diagnosed with cancer in 2011.[4] According to the Cancer Prevention Coalition, from 1950 to 1995 the overall increase of all cancers rose 55%.[5] Governments brag about the increased cure rate of cancer, but this focus masks the brutal reality that although survival rates may be better, the number of newly diagnosed cases is alarming. Perhaps most alarming is the incidence of cancer in children, which has risen almost 30% in the past 20 years.[6]

Diabetes. In 2011, 25.8 million people in the US were diagnosed with diabetes. That is 8.3% of the population and doesn't account for the millions of Americans that go undiagnosed. In 2010, 26.9 percent of US residents age 65 years or older had diabetes. In just the four years from 2008 to 2012 diabetes rates increased 9 percent![7] As is the case with cancer, childhood diabetes has seen dramatic increases over the past 20 years. Although consistent statistics seem hard to find, reputable sources seem to agree that it is a frightening problem. The CDC website states, "In the last 2 decades, type 2 diabetes (formerly known as adult-onset diabetes) has been reported among U.S. children and adolescents with increasing frequency."[8]

"The changing demography of childhood diabetes has major implications for our understanding of

---

[4] http://seer.cancer.gov/statfacts/html/all.html
[5] http://www.preventcancer.com/losing/nci/manipulates.htm
[6] http://www.cancer.gov/cancertopics/factsheet/Sites-Types/childhood
[7] http://www.huffingtonpost.com/2011/01/26/diabetes-rates-in-america-_n_814432.html
[8] http://www.cdc.gov/diabetes/projects/cda2.htm

the disease. A rapid change in incidence within a genetically stable population implies that non-genetic factors are active and that the influence of genes is relative to population, time, and place. It suggests that something has changed in the environment our children encounter or in the way they are reared."[9]

Cardiovascular disease. In 2008, heart disease was the leading cause of death for both men and women in the United States. Although it is hard to know exactly how many Americans might have heart disease, data from the CDC's Behavioral Risk Factor Surveillance System found that in 2010 approximately 6% of the population reported heart disease of some kind. The incidence of death due to heart related problems has declined because of early detection technologies, but the age that heart disease is being detected is earlier and earlier. One report shows that signs of heart disease in sedentary children are being detected as early as 6-9 years of age.

More diseases on the rise

Cancer, diabetes, and heart disease have all been around for a long time and don't seem so shocking to the average person. However, it's not just chronic illnesses that are on the rise: there are all kinds of different illnesses—many of which most of us had never heard of prior to ten or fifteen years ago.

---

[9] http://diabetes.diabetesjournals.org/content/51/12/3353.full

ADD/ADHD. The American Psychiatric Society created the name Attention Deficit Disorder in 1980. Basically, it was a term coined for children who exhibited impulsive behaviors. In 1987, the name was revised to Attention Deficit Hyperactivity Disorder. According to the CDC, rates of ADHD diagnosis increased an average of 3% per year from 1997 to 2003 and 5.5% per year from 2003 to 2007.[10] Perhaps what is even more alarming is that the percentage of children with a parent-reported ADHD diagnosis increased by 22% between 2003 and 2007. Although adults are diagnosed with this condition, its rapid growth exists primarily in children. This makes it difficult for statisticians and medical professionals to say that life-expectancy is the cause of such a high growth trend.

Autism. According to the CDC, Autism Spectrum Disorder (ASD) rates among U.S. children almost doubled between the years of 2002 and 2008, going from 6.6 out of 1,000 children to 11.3. Once again, life expectancy has no impact on these childhood disease increases.

It's not just chronic illnesses that are on the rise: there are all kinds of different illnesses—many of which most of us had never heard of prior to ten or fifteen years ago.

---

[10] http://www.cdc.gov/ncbddd/adhd/data.html

Thyroid. Talk to any woman over the age of 40 and she'll know someone—if not herself—who has been diagnosed with either an underactive (the more common) or overactive thyroid. The main function of the thyroid gland is to produce, store, and emit two different thyroid hormones: thyroxin and triodothyronine. Thyroid dysfunction is due to either increased or decreased emission of the thyroid hormones. According to the National Thyroid Institute, "the rate of metabolism in the body is regulated by the thyroid hormones, as is heat production and oxygen utilization. Thyroid hormones also provide the specific proteins to different organs and tissues. Due of the importance of all this, problems with the thyroid gland can have a very significant effect to the body."[11]

A low metabolism means that the body is burning fewer calories than normal, which often results in weight gain—even when the individual modifies caloric input and increases exercise participation. Currently 68% of Americans are overweight or clinically obese. Some believe there is a direct link between thyroid disease and obesity. Others believe it is environmental conditions affecting the thyroid that are causing the increase. Whatever is the blame, thyroid disease is a fast rising trend.

Fibromyalgia. Fibromyalgia is now a common syndrome in which a person has long-term, body-wide pain and tenderness in the joints, muscles, tendons, and other soft tissues. The medical term fibromyalgia was coined in

---

[11] http://www.nationalthyroidinstitute.org/thyroid-disorders/

1976; the first controlled clinical study with validation of known symptoms and tender points was published in 1981.[12] Although statistics on the historical numbers of fibromyalgia were not readily available, it seems the numbers are sizable when pharmaceutical companies are televising ads about treatment with drugs like Lyrica. These companies wouldn't spend millions of dollars on ads during peak viewing times without knowing they have market share to win over.

Although the term fibromyalgia wasn't used until 1976, research implies that the condition has been around for decades. Why was it that you never heard of so many people having this intensely debilitating pain until recently? Skeptics say it's because the disease went undiagnosed, but for many health care professionals that argument just doesn't hold up.

The list goes on and on. Irritable bowel syndrome, depression, celiac and/or gluten intolerance, heartburn, indigestion, and leaky gut syndrome are just a few of the more common. These are diseases that, until recently, have never been heard of by most people. Yet, in our respective wellness practices in the U.S. and Australia, these diseases are all too common. Even seemingly healthy people who eat well and exercise regularly show disturbing signs of "dis-ease". It's alarming.

Take a minute now and reflect upon your friends, family members, and co-workers. Does it seem to you that

---

[12] http://www.ncbi.nlm.nih.gov/pubmed/15361321

more and more people are getting sick? Certainly we are not implying that everyone is walking around with life-threatening diseases, but rather the vast majority is displaying signs that their body is not functioning well. Things like poor sleep patterns, anxiety, skin rashes, hives, and frequent colds or allergies that don't seem to go away. These may not be diseases or serious illnesses, but they indicate a weakened immune system.

The question many natural health practitioners and wellness advocates are asking is, "Why, in this modern age of medical technology and unlimited supply of cutting-edge drugs and treatments, are we seemingly getting weaker, and not stronger and healthier?" To answer that, let's move onto a discussion about what affects our health.

"Why, in this modern age of medical technology and unlimited supply of cutting-edge drugs and treatments, are we seemingly getting weaker, and not stronger and healthier?"

Chapter 1

The Components of Good Health

The components of good health are pretty basic; good air (oxygen), good water, good food, good sleep and good exercise. Regardless of what science tells us, your body intuitively knows that these basic elements are necessary to maintain health.

Think about how you feel when you go out on a hike in the woods, skiing in the mountains, or spend time at a remote beachfront. Most people get out into the fresh air, take a deep breath, and respond audibly, "ahhhh, smell that air!" Similarly, remember back to a time you exercised and became really thirsty. You didn't reach for a cup of coffee; your body was calling for water and it quenched your thirst and tasted great—even though it has no taste. Whether it is the sweet delight of a freshly cut watermelon, the refreshed feeling you have upon waking up after an uninterrupted, no-alarm-clock-needed sleep, or the energy you exude after a workout—your body and mind respond positively when you give it any of these desirable components.

Although mankind once had fresh air, water, food, rest when the sun went down (no electricity), and high levels of physical activity as a way of life, these environmental conditions no longer exist.

Good air

Unless you live in some remote area of the world that has not been inhabited by houses, factories, and cars, the air most people breathe is polluted. Car exhaust and industrial emissions alone are more than enough to cause outdoor air pollution. Add to this all the indoor pollutants that eventually end up outdoors and it makes things worse. Think of all the chemicals in our world that emit gases: household cleaners, spray paints, fabric treatments, pesticides, and herbicides, just to name a few. All of these types of products "off-gas" into the environment and into the air we breathe every day—in our home, our car and outdoors.

Good water

Water makes up a high percentage of all your body's cells. Humans can survive more than a month without food but only a few days without water. A hydrated body is a healthy body, but what happens when the water we consume contains contaminants; some you can taste and some which you can't, like heavy metals? Although the answer is obvious, let's use a simple example to emphasize the point. Take a healthy plant and begin to add toxic chemicals to the water you provide it; it will slowly die. Sure, it may "adapt" for some time, but eventually with enough toxicity it will die.

To say that the quality of the water most people drink is less than perfect would be an understatement. Due to air pollution, marine dumping, industrial waste, radioactive waste, and human waste, there are very few "natural" sources of water, if any. You may be thinking, "but that's okay, I drink town or city water that has been treated, so it's safe." Most public water supplies, however, are recycled from wastewater; chlorine and fluoride are added along with as many as 171 other chemicals that are supposedly safe. Yet, even with all the treatments and chemicals, you often hear of towns announcing "boil the water before drinking" because bacteria levels are dangerously high. But boiling water only kills viruses; it does not remove heavy metals and other dissolved solids.

Good food

The human body needs food to survive, but it needs good food to thrive. So, what is good food? The answer to that will be different depending upon whom you ask. Ask a typical 16 year-old teenager and he might say, "A 3-piece combo special from Kentucky Fried Chicken all washed down with a Mountain Dew." Ask a nutritionist and you'll get something more along the lines of "a calorically balanced meal of lean protein, fresh fruits and vegetables, and an all natural complex carbohydrate like quinoa."

The reality of today's food supply is scary. Most people in the Western world eat an enormous amount of pre-packaged foods, fast food and restaurant meals multiple days a week, and consume high volumes of beverages other than water. There is an alarming number of sugary soft drinks, high calorie, fat-latent coffee drinks and chemically packed "energy" drinks with ingredients you can't pronounce.

Colors, preservatives, additives, sugar, and hydrogenated fats are so common in the average person's diet that many have to think about the last time they had a meal that was completely "natural," meaning that nothing was taken from a package before eating.

If you were born before 1964, you may remember growing up with a grocery store that had just a few "snack" options. Nuts, pretzels, and potato chips were what your mother would bring home. A bag of chips was 6 oz., and one bag would be bought for an entire family to share. Today's grocery store has an entire double-sided aisle dedicated only to chip products. A 5.5oz. or 155g bag is now considered the "snack size" with some "family size" bags weighing in at 2 pounds or 900g! So, not only has the number of high fat, high sugar, and high sodium products exploded, most of them also come in larger and larger sizes. It's no wonder that both the US and Australia are among the countries with the highest obesity rates worldwide!

Good sleep

According to the CDC:

> "Sleep is being increasingly recognized as important to public health. Insufficient sleep

is linked to motor vehicle crashes, industrial accidents and disasters and medical and other occupational errors. People who suffer from sleep insufficiency are also more likely to suffer from chronic diseases such as hypertension, diabetes, depression and obesity, as well as from cancer, increased mortality, and reduced quality of life and productivity."[13]

There are many different types of sleep disorders—from things as common as snoring and anxiety, to more severe disorders like sleep apnea or restless leg syndrome. All in all, there are 85 different documented sleep disorders that currently affect almost 20% of the US population.[14] Sleep disorders certainly aren't new, but the number of adults and children who report having sleep difficulties is rising. In addition to the constant go-go and stress of everyday life, many believe that the increase in sleep issues has risen in direct proportion to technological advancements. Let's face it—we rarely "unplug." You once went on vacation and couldn't be reached except through a hotel phone, but now you have a phone on your hip 24-7, and it can send and receive e-mails and text messages. Add things like Facebook, YouTube, and Twitter, and it is easy to see how people are so distracted with communication that their sleep suffers.

Physiologically, the body *and* the mind need rest. It is during our sleep that our bodies restore and regenerate.

---

[13] http://www.cdc.gov/Features/dsSleep/
[14] http://4mind4life.com/blog/2010/07/30/sleep-disorder-statistics/

Most people don't know that there are actually 5 stages of sleep: relaxation, light sleep, two stages of deep sleep called delta sleep, and finally REM, or the rapid eye movement stage. The body goes through cycles of these stages throughout the night. If we don't sleep enough hours, we won't get enough cycles. If sleep is interrupted the cycles are broken, hence incomplete. In either instance, our bodies do not regenerate, and we awake feeling sluggish, tired, and even grumpy. Continued sleep disturbances can lead to exhaustion, depression and ultimately contribute to chronic diseases.

Good exercise

When you visualize a healthy person, you probably imagine someone who is fit, not flabby or fat. Certainly, they don't need to have bulging muscles, but there is something very attractive about a man with a well-defined upper body or a woman whose toned shoulders and arms are shown off in a sleeveless shirt.

Decades ago, our grandparents got plenty of exercise in their daily lives. Cars were a luxury, and people walked places and rode bicycles. Prior to a washing machine clothes had to be hand scrubbed and rung out to dry. Bread consumptions involved mixing and kneading—not just running to the grocery store! And consider the task of ironing before electricity: one had to warm a heavy iron over a fire and then, while it was hot, iron quickly.

Today, our lives are full of conveniences, and the incidental exercise we get from daily activities is very minimal, if any. We use escalators and stairs, drive everywhere, put clothes into a washing machine and electric dryer, and buy fruits and vegetables instead of growing them. Many jobs consist of sitting or using automation to perform heavy lifting or moving and, at the end of the day we sit in front of a television where we don't even have to get up to find hundreds of channels. Most live sedentary lives—even kids who, instead of going outside to run and play, sit in front of computers, X-box and smart phones, which is an ironic name when you think about it.

The result of a sedentary society is clear to the eye and costly. The most recent statistics by the CDC report that the number of Americans that are either overweight or clinically obese is 68%. The annual cost of obesity in 2008 was $147 billion and climbing. However, the most alarming is the obesity rates among children. In 2009, 17% of US children ages 2-19 were obese (not just overweight). Since 1980, obesity prevalence among children and adolescents has almost tripled.[15]

On a more positive note, it is estimated that 80% of all chronic illnesses in western societies can be prevented with regular exercise. With a combination of moderate levels of cardiovascular (aerobic) and strength training (anaerobic) exercise, individuals can maintain good health and fitness.

---

[15] www.cdc.gov/obesity/childhood/data.html

27

Aerobic exercise increases the body's ability to use oxygen. That, in turn, helps to improve the function of the heart and lungs, resulting in the body having the ability to pump more blood per minute. Oxygen is the life force; more oxygen means better health. Improved cardiovascular functions can also mean lower blood pressure. There are many other positive effects, but these alone are significant.

Anaerobic exercise, commonly referred to as strength training, is also a critical component of a balanced exercise program. By exercising ones' muscles, not only does it result in greater strength, but it also helps to maintain strong tendons and ligaments as well as positively impacting bone density. When combined with a healthy diet, those who strength-train have a lower body fat percentage, a better metabolism, and improved glucose tolerance and insulin sensitivity. Improved coordination, balance, and functional ability are additional benefits for older adults to help in fall prevention.

Many people don't realize that the benefits of exercise can be obtained with moderate participation. Two days a week of strength training for 15 minutes and three days a week of getting at least 30 minutes of cardiovascular training will help maintain good health throughout life. And we always tell people to keep it in perspective; any amount of exercise each week is better than none! A big reason many do not do enough physical activity (or any) is that they are carrying excess weight, don't feel well, lack energy, or suffer muscular, joint, and back pain.

Are we in control?

It goes without saying that each of these components to good health—air, water, food, sleep, and exercise are not exclusive of one another. You can drink clean water, eat organic food, get plenty of sleep and exercise, and still die from lung cancer because you were exposed to asbestos at some stage in your life. It is the combination of all these things throughout your life that have an impact.

What is concerning to so many people in the holistic field is the reality that, no matter how careful you try to be, you can't control everything. Sure, you could check out of society, go to the most remote but habitable part of the world, and live off the land, and probably stay incredibly healthy from a physical perspective. But, since you would be living by yourself it might be a bit lonely and emotionally stressful!

Even if you have an air purifier in your home, a household water purification system, and eat organic, you still have to

---

It goes without saying that each of these components to good health—air, water, food, sleep, and exercise are not exclusive of one another.

---

function in society. You are being exposed to air pollution, treated water, and pesticides. <u>The key is to manage as much of it as you can as often as you can</u>. Continually educate yourself on the best choices and strategies for each of the five components—air, water, food, sleep and exercise—and you will feel better knowing that you are giving yourself the best possible chance to be healthy.

Chapter 2

Hidden Dangers You MUST Know About

In the section discussing good air, water, and food, we identified environmental and industrial pollution, chlorine, fluoride, pesticides, and preservatives as just some of the potentially dangerous substances you are inhaling and consuming every day. However, there are two other categories of substances that are incredibly dangerous to humans: synthetic fragrances and dyes, and petrochemicals. The substances in these categories are most often found in personal care products and household cleaners, and although we are not eating them, we are 'consuming' them through our bodies by either topical application or contact when using a product around the home. Before we get into the specific dangers of these substances, let's first discuss how your skin works.

How your skin works

Although most people don't think of it as such, your skin is an organ. In fact, it is the largest organ of your body, making up around 16% of your total body weight. Skin replenishes itself at a rate of about 30,000 to 40,000 cells a minute, which means you replace roughly nine pounds (4.1) kilograms of skin each year.[16]

Skin has four major functions: protection, insulation, temperature regulation, and sensation. It protects us by acting as a barrier between what is under the skin and the environment that we live in. It is also our body's first line of defense against diseases and parasites. It insulates our body while also acting as a thermostat by being able to alter the blood vessel diameter of your skin. If you are cold, the dermal blood vessels constrict so heat loss is minimized and you warm up. If you are hot, they do the opposite and open up, allowing your body to vent and cool down. Skin also conducts sensation, both alerting you to danger and allowing you to enjoy touch.

Skin has three distinct layers: the epidermis, which is the outermost layer of the skin and provides a waterproof barrier; the dermis, which contains tough connective tissue, hair follicles, and sweat glands; and the hypodermis, which is the deeper subcutaneous tissue that is made up of fat and connective tissue.

Here's the important (and scary) part

Anything you put on your skin gets absorbed into your body. Once it penetrates the epidermis, it enters the hair follicles (also known as pores) and sweat glands and

---

[16] http://health.howstuffworks.com/skin-care/information/anatomy/function-of-skin.htm

eventually works its way into the deeper tissues and into your blood stream. Therefore, if you put anything toxic on your skin it could have a negative affect on your body. Even chlorine and other chemicals in our water system get to our skin in our daily shower and also in the air that we inhale.

The effects of these toxins might not happen immediately, but eventually if you take in more toxins than the body can process and excrete, it begins to pollute your body. This is the same process that occurs when pesticides are used on crops—eventually the runoff from the soil reaches the rivers, lakes, and oceans and results in polluted water.

The skull & crossbones history

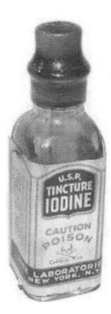

Do you remember when certain products had skull and crossbones on the bottle? That label meant that the product was considered poisonous. If you are from the Baby Boomer generation you will remember this, but if you were born after 1970 you probably don't because packaging didn't have the symbol on it anymore. You might be wondering, "What happened to these products? Were they taken off the market?" The answer is NO.

In 1980, the big chemical companies petitioned the US Government and Congress and said something like, "We

33

are having a tough time selling our household and personal use products to Moms because some of the ingredients require us to put this scary skull and crossbones on the bottle. We'd like to propose a new labeling system that will be better."

As you might suspect, the petition succeeded and now millions of products that would have previously required a skull and crossbones logo on the package are sitting on the shelves of your home. Most people aren't even aware of this change (and the companies making a fortune on these products are glad of it). Instead of the skull and crossbones needing to be used, one of three words must appear on the package: "**Danger**," "**Warning**," or "**Caution**."

As you read those words you might be saying to yourself, "Oh, yea, now that you mention it I can recall seeing those." You should, because they appear on just about every product you buy from a standard grocery store, home improvement store, or discount chain.

What this means to you is the following: <u>If any of these words appear on a product in your home, that package would have required a skull and crossbones prior to 1980.</u>

Now millions of products that would have previously required a skull and crossbones logo on the package are sitting on the shelves of your home.

Perhaps even more alarming are the thresholds that meet the requirements of each of those labels.

- Danger = 1 taste to 1 tsp can be fatal to an adult.
- Warning = 1 tsp to an oz. can be fatal to an adult.
- Caution = 1 oz. to a pint of water can be fatal to an adult.

Whether the product is designated as a Danger, Warning or Caution, the words that follow it are the scariest: *"Harmful or fatal if absorbed by or through the skin, ingested or inhaled."* These thresholds are for an adult. Imagine how little it takes to be harmful to an infant, or small, growing children.

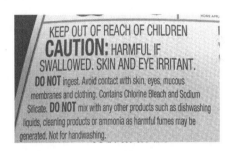

KEEP OUT OF REACH OF CHILDREN

CAUTION: HARMFUL IF SWALLOWED. SKIN AND EYE IRRITANT.

DO NOT ingest. Avoid contact with skin, eyes, mucous membranes and clothing. Contains Chlorine Bleach and Sodium Silicate. DO NOT mix with any other products such as dishwashing liquids, cleaning products or ammonia as harmful fumes may be generated. Not for handwashing.

Danger categories

There are a total of 8 categories of products that the 1980 packaging laws affected. In alphabetical order they are: alcohols, chlorines, detergents & emulsifiers, heavy metals, pesticides, petrochemicals, preservatives, and synthetic fragrances & dyes. The three most prevalent in households are synthetic fragrances and dyes, petrochemicals, and preservatives.

Synthetic fragrances

Synthetic fragrances are exactly what they say—smells that have been synthetically manufactured with the use of chemicals in a laboratory. They are commonly found in personal care products such as lotions, shaving products, deodorants, and perfumes, to name a few. What is inconceivable is that packaging laws do not require manufacturers to disclose what ingredients are used to make their 'fragrance' because it is considered a trade secret! Therefore, for anything that has the word "fragrance" in the ingredient list, you have absolutely no idea what has been put into it. Whatever it is, it is chemically created, which is why, according to a University of West Georgia study, as many as 30% of people surveyed reported sensitivity and irritation to scented products.[17]

An ingredient that is often hidden in a products fragrance trade secret is phthalates. Phthalates (pronounced "thah-lates") are chemical plasticizers that have been widely used since the 1950's as a softening agent. In personal care items, they're used to help lubricate other substances,

---

What is inconceivable is that packaging laws do not require manufacturers to disclose what ingredients are used to make their 'fragrance' because it is considered a trade secret!

---

[17] http://www.everydayhealth.com/allergies/fragrance-sensitivity.aspx

help lotions penetrate and soften the skin, and help fragrances last longer.[18] ALL phthalates are banned in Europe, but the U.S. regulations allow companies to knowingly include them into products under the protection of their "trade secrets!"

Synthetic fragrances and dyes that are documented to have the following side effects include:[19]

- Allergic reactions
- Muscular aches and pains
- Vertigo
- Emotional behavioral problems
- Oral tumors
- Dizziness
- Upset stomach
- Convulsions
- Reproductive problems

- Skin rashes
- Coughing
- Hyperactivity
- Leukemia
- Organ damage
- Depression
- Sneezing
- ADD
- Cancer

Following is a short list of products that your family is probably exposed to and that have known dangerous chemical compounds in them. Household cleaners were added as a "category", but not separately listed because if we had to list all the various kinds it would take up too much space!

- Air fresheners
- Bath soap

- Toothpaste medication
- Nail polish

---

[18] http://www.babycenter.ca/baby/safety/phthalates/
[19] Get a Whiff of This; Perfumes (fragrances)—the Invisible Chemical Poisons, Connie Pitts

- Shower gel
- Bubble bath
- Hair shampoo
- Skin lotion
- After shave
- Cologne or perfume
- Acne medication
- Hand sanitizer
- Hair spray
- Dry cleaning

- Hair gel
- Laundry detergent
- Hair conditioners
- Mouthwash
- Facial cleaners
- All household cleaners
- Deodorant
- Fabric softener
- Cosmetics

You may be saying to yourself, "Wait a minute; the Government wouldn't allow these chemicals in our products if they weren't safe for us." In her book, *Dying to Look Good*, Christine Farlow, D.C., noted:

"The cosmetics industry is very poorly regulated. The Federal Food, Drug, and Cosmetic (FD&C) Act does not require cosmetics and personal care products or their ingredients to be approved before they are marketed and sold to consumers. FDA regulation starts *after* they are already in the marketplace. So, except for color additives and a few ingredients, which are banned, manufacturers may use whatever ingredients they choose in the cosmetics and personal care products they produce without approval from the FDA. . . . The FDA can make suggestions or recommendations to manufacturers about cosmetic products or their ingredients, but *the manufacturers do not have to comply*. The FDA must first prove in a court of law that a product is harmful, improperly labeled, or violates the law if it wants to remove a cosmetic product from the market."[20]

She goes on to quote John Bailey, Ph.D., who at one time was the director of the FDA'S Office of Cosmetics and Colors as saying, "Consumers believe that 'if it's on the market, it can't hurt me,' and this belief is sometimes wrong."

Petrochemicals

The second extremely dangerous category of products we need to discuss is petrochemicals. Petrochemicals are chemicals made from petroleum (crude oil) and natural gas. There are over **4,000** products classified as "*petrochemicals*", many of which are not used at all in personal care and household products. But, there is a handful that is used in almost every product out there and they alone are incredibly dangerous. Let's discuss each of them.

Diethanolamine

Commonly abbreviated as DEA, this product belongs to a class of chemicals known as alkanolamines. DEA and two other chemicals in this class (monoethanolamine or MEA) and triethanolamine or **TEA**), "**have** been linked with kidney, liver, and other organ damage according to several government-funded research studies, and has been proven to cause cancer in rats when applied to the skin.

---

[20] Dying to Look Good, Christine Hoza Farlow, D.C., 2nd Edition, 2006, p. 17 & 18

According to a 1995 study funded by the <u>National Institute of Environmental Health Sciences</u>, **DEA** has low acute toxicity but significant cumulative toxicity. This is because it cannot be easily excreted from the body but instead **builds up** in the fatty tissues of the liver, brain, kidneys, and spleen with repeated oral and dermal exposure."[21]

Propylene glycol

Aso called Propanediol or abbreviated PEG, propylene glycol is a colorless, viscous, hygroscopic liquid used in anti-freeze, brake and hydraulic fluid, paints and coatings, and de-icer. It also keeps products from melting in heat and freezing when it is cold.

Did we mention that it's also in the lotions, deodorants, and cosmetics most of us put on our bodies because it acts as a penetration enhancer? That's right; this is not an error or typo. The primary ingredient in anti-freeze is often one of the most prevalent ingredients in personal care products. Not a nice thought, is it?

Here's what is so controversial: The FDA allows propylene glycol to be added into personal care products, but the Environmental Protection Agency (EPA) warns factory workers to avoid skin contact with propylene glycol to prevent brain, liver, and kidney abnormalities. And if you think that we are talking about just a few products or negligible amounts, think again.

---

[21] http://thomko.squarespace.com/dangers-of-dea/

Propylene glycol is in thousands of personal care products for one primary reason—money. Oh, sure, PEG does accomplish what the manufacturers want by helping their products to penetrate the skin, but the truth is that it is cheap, acts as a filler, and keeps the cost of manufacturing lower.

For big companies, it is all about the bottom line. Cigarette manufacturers, drug companies, and dozens of other corporations have continued to produce and sell dangerous products--even when they know it has harmful side effects—simply to make money and keep investors happy. Those not believing this are simply naïve. Sure, we are believers in capitalism, so long as it is socially responsible.

Sodium lauryl sulfate

A third chemical we need to alert you about is Sodium Lauryl Sulfate, also called Sodium Laureth Sulfate and abbreviated SLS or SLES. SLS is the primary ingredient in engine degreasers but manufacturers add SLS to personal care products to create a foaming action.

The FDA allows propylene glycol to be added into personal care products, but the Environmental Protection Agency (EPA) warns factory workers to avoid skin contact with propylene glycol to prevent brain, liver, and kidney abnormalities.

In the same way that it dissolves grease on car engines, SLS removes grease from your skin and hair, which can actually cause a drying effect—i.e. damaged or frizzy hair and dry, itchy skin, or ezcema like symptoms. This drying can change your skin's PH, thereby increasing the risk of infections.

"In its final report on the safety of sodium lauryl sulfate, the *Journal of the American College of Toxicology* notes that this ingredient has a 'degenerative effect on the cell membranes because of its protein denaturing properties.' What's more, the journal adds, 'high levels of skin penetration may occur at even low use concentration.'"[22]

Like propylene glycol, manufacturers use SLS because: a. it accomplishes the desired action of foaming so consumers feel like the product is working, and, b. it's cheap.

The real cost

Although the cost to purchase products with DEA, PEG and SLS might be cheap, the potential cost to your health isn't. Here is a list of the known side effects of these petrochemicals:

• Inhibit skin growth	• Pimples
• Sensitivity to sun	• Headaches
• Fatigue	• Respiratory problems
• Immune system disorders	• Rashes
• Depression	• Reproductive disorders

---

[22] http://www.natural-health-information-centre.com/sodium-lauryl-sulfate.html

We realize for many people reading this book the realization that many of the products they use daily could be toxic can be too much to comprehend at first glance. We don't expect you to believe us at face value. We encourage you to go online and do your own research.

Even if you come across a site that tells you small doses of these chemicals are perfectly safe, you need to ask yourself these questions:

1. Who is responsible for the content on the site? Is it a governmental site or perhaps something sponsored by a manufacturer of products that use these chemicals?
2. What are the cumulative effects? That is, what happens when you are using many, many products each day that all have a little bit of these chemicals in them?
3. What are the levels that can be tolerated by infants, small children and household pets?

We can't answer those questions for you. You will need to come to your own conclusions. What we can do is recommend that you take greater control of your environment and what you put into and on your body (and your family members too).

We suggest that you take out all your personal care and household cleaning products, sit down next to your computer and begin to Google the listed ingredients. Educate yourself so you can make totally informed decisions for you and your family.

Some good news

At this point in the book you might be thinking to yourself, "Wait a minute; the title of this book is Vibrant Health Now and everything I've read up to now is downright depressing!" We are absolutely going to get to that information; it's just that this information is necessary as a backdrop to understanding the suggestions that will be made.

Further, there is good news; YOU HAVE A CHOICE! Hopefully, this book will provide you with valuable insights that will motivate you to start a healthier journey and rid your household and your life of dangerous products that you may have unknowingly been using every day.

We suggest that you take out all your personal care and household cleaning products, sit down next to your computer and begin to Google the listed ingredients.

Chapter 3

How Chemicals Affect Your Body

Now that you know about the various products and substances that are dangerous, the next logical question is, "Okay, so these substances are toxic, but exactly how are they actually affecting my body?" Let's face it, you may be completely healthy and/or you may not have associated any of your current health situations to everyday product usage. To answer this, we need to have a small lesson on the molecular structure of the human body.

Your body is made up of many things. Tissue, bones, organs and blood are terms that we are all familiar with, but each of those is actually made up of trillions of cells. Scientists estimate that the human body has between 75 and 100 trillion cells.

Cells provide structure and stability as well as energy, yet they cannot be seen without magnification. They contain DNA, which is genetic information necessary for directing cellular activities. They also contain structures called organelles, which have a wide range of responsibilities and carry out specific functions within a cell, including providing the energy necessary to produce hormones and enzymes. They group together and form tissue; tissue groups together to form organs. And, cells reproduce by cloning themselves and they vary in lifespan from days to as much as a year.[23] Those are the basics.

The cell 'city'

Alan uses a great analogy for how cells work. He first heard a version of this from Dr. Bruce Lipton, an internationally recognized speaker and author of The Biology of Belief.

Imagine that every cell is like its own self-contained city. For a city to function well, there are many things that need to happen every single day. The city needs electricity (or power), homes and businesses for people to live and work in, workers in every profession (including politicians), cars and other mass transportation, running water, clean food supplies, trash pick up, etc. If anyone of these functions stops working or slows down, the entire city suffers. Think of how quickly a city has problems when the trash collectors go on strike!

In addition to normal, everyday functions, a city is always concerned about the safety of its people. If the city comes under attack, people are told to take cover and prepare for potential danger. When this happens, people go indoors, sometimes even taking refuge in bunkers if the threat is

---

[23] http://biology.about.com/od/cellbiology/a/cells-facts.htm

significant enough. As a result, everything on the city's surface comes to a screeching halt—no building, no repair, no business, no trash collection, etc.

Furthermore, people are forced to live off of the supplies they have stored away. For short periods of time this is a manageable situation, but if people have to stay underground for any length of time sickness and disease will occur.

The goal in providing you with this very simple explanation is singular. You must understand that if your cells are not able to function in a "normal, everyday environment," your body will not function optimally. If your body is under constant attack from toxins—bad air, bad water, bad food, poor sleep, extended periods of stress, topical and inhaled chemicals, etc.—your cells cannot maintain optimal health.

Damaged cells are attacked by healthy cells in an effort to heal. Although the body is doing what it needs, this process can trigger inflammation and is likely a contributor to the development of auto immune diseases today. In some instances cells mutate into things like tumors.

You must understand that if your cells are not able to function in a "normal, everyday environment," your body will not function optimally.

Regardless of the degree of damage, weak, damaged, or mutated cells continue to clone themselves (remember this is how they reproduce). The result will be a body in state of "dis-ease" and this can eventually, and often does, lead to disease.

Conversely, if we do things to maintain vibrant cells we will be more likely to stay healthy. <u>Therefore, the critical question becomes, "What can I do to maintain cellular vitality?"</u>

Cellular vitality & frequency

By taking our discussion of cells even deeper, we learn that every cell has molecules, which have protons and electrons that are constantly in motion. (We promise, that is as detailed as we will get!). The result of this activity is an electromagnetic field, or force field of energy that each cell emits. This "field" is often depicted in sci-fi and super hero movies, but it is an actual reality of the body, and there are various imaging cameras and devices that can photograph a person's electromagnetic field.

One way of measuring cellular energy is by measuring electromagnetic frequency. Every electrical thing has a frequency that can be measured in hertz (Hz).

The late Bruce Tanio, who was head of the Department of Agriculture at Eastern Washington University, in Washington State, developed a Calibrated Frequency Monitor (CFM) to measure frequencies of plants.

Specifically, Mr. Tanio used the CFM to measure the frequencies of humans, foods, essential oils and disease. Here is what he found:

A healthy human body has a frequency range from 62-68MHz (brain goes higher). When holding a cup of coffee one man's frequency dropped from 66 to 58MHz in just 3 seconds. It took three days for that man's frequency to return to normal. A second man drank the coffee and his frequency dropped from 66 to 52MHz. In another case, a man held a cigarette and his frequency dropped from 65 to 48MHz, and upon smoking, it went down to 42.[24]

Here are some other interesting things he discovered with this testing:[25]

- A healthy human brain is between 71-90 MHz (mega hertz)
- When you have cold symptoms your frequency drops to 58 MHz.
- When you have a Candida infection your frequency is 55 MHz.

A healthy human body has a frequency range from 62-68MHz.

---

[24] http://www.webdeb.com/oils/frequency.htm
[25] The Chemistry of Essential Oils, David Stewart, Ph.D., D.N.M., 2006, p. 182

- When you have Epstein Barr syndrome your frequency is 52 MHz.
- When you have cancer your frequency is 42 MHz.
- When you begin to die your frequency is 25 MHz.
- Processed or canned foods have a frequency of 0 (zero) MHz.
- Depending upon how fresh, produce ranges in frequency between 10-15 MHz.
- Fresh herbs have a frequency between 20-27 MHz.
- Dry herbs have a frequency between 12-22 MHz.

Another very interesting thing Tanio discovered with his device is how thought influences the effects on the human body. We all have been in a situation where a "downer" friend meets us for lunch and, upon getting away from them, you think to yourself, "Wow, just being around them makes me feel lousy." Well, Tanio discovered that this isn't just a psychological feeling, but an actual physical effect.

Specifically, he found that negative thoughts lowered a person's frequency by 12 MHz. This quantification of energetic decrease really gives new meaning to the saying, "If you want to fly with the eagles, don't hang with the turkeys." If you hang around people who have bad attitudes or are negative, don't be surprised if you begin to feel badly yourself!

Negative thoughts lowered a person's frequency by 12 MHz.

On a more positive note Tanio also discovered that the opposite held true to a lesser extent. That is, a positive thought raised a person's frequency by 10 MHz. What is particularly curious about this is the fact that negative thoughts actually have more energy to them than positive ones. This is probably where the expression "one bad apple can spoil the whole bunch" came from. It was also found that prayer and meditation increased frequency levels by 15 MHz.[26]

Here's THE kicker

What we haven't shared with you yet is perhaps the most interesting discovery of Tanio's research. Remember the coffee example? Upon drinking the beverage, the man's frequency dropped from 66MHz to 52MHz. *Here's the amazing part: the Eastern Washington University researchers had the man who drank the coffee inhale an essential oil blend[27] and his frequency returned to 66 in just 21 seconds!*

Stated another way, with only the inhalation of a therapeutic grade essential oil the man's frequency went from 52MHz, where Epstein Barr can manifest, back to 66MHz, which is a totally healthy frequency. This is the incredible power of authentic therapeutic grade essential oils.

Notice our emphasis on "authentic therapeutic grade." In a later section we will be discussing more about the various

---

[26] The Chemistry of Essential Oils, David Stewart, Ph.D., D.N.M., 2006, p. 183
[27] The blend of oil that was used was Young Living "R.C."

grades of oils and why it is absolutely imperative that you are using only authentic therapeutic grade oils for health and well being. But for now let's get back to our discussion of frequency.

A frequency distinction

Earlier we noted that all things have a frequency that can be measured. An important distinction (especially for those science-minded individuals) is the difference between coherent and incoherent frequencies, as they relate to your body and your health.

To keep it simple, vibration puts off sound waves. Some sound waves are in a form we can hear, but many we do not. Whether or not we hear a frequency doesn't change the fact that it has an impact on our energy field (remember how thoughts impacted frequency). But in addition to the strength of a frequency, the type of frequency also has an impact.

As the name implies, incoherent (also referred to as chaotic) frequencies generate waves that would be equivalent to a game of *Asteroids* against your force field, shooting varying waves that interrupt your energy. In fact,

---

With only the inhalation of a therapeutic grade essential oil the man's frequency went from 52MHz, where Epstein Barr can manifest, back to 66MHz.

---

incoherent frequencies are known to fracture the human electrical field and can interfere with human DNA.

For example, lights and other electrical appliances are 60Hz in the U.S. and 50HZ in Australia and work off of alternating current (AC). If you didn't know the difference between incoherent and coherent you might conclude that lights would have no impact on a person's frequency. However, lights and electrical appliances are incoherent. This explains why so many people complain of headaches when around fluorescent lighting!

Coherent, or harmonic frequencies are just the opposite; they do not fracture the human electrical field. As you might have suspected, essential oils have a coherent, harmonic frequency so they are harmonious with the electrical field of the human body.

High frequency = high health

At this point in our discussion, we hope you have come to realize that the concept of frequency as it relates to your health and well-being is critical. Frequency is energy and, when your energy is high, the cells are vibrating at such a rate that your force field is strong. Literally a high-vibrational frequency creates a force field around you. In this state, bacteria and viruses are kept at bay.

Therefore, the key to maintaining health is rooted in maintaining a high personal frequency.

Everything you do in a day—every choice of food and beverage you put into your body, every product that you put onto your body, every thought you allow into your head, every situation you find yourself in, EVERYTHING impacts your frequency level or force field. Said as simply as possible:

Positive choices = improved frequency
Negative choices = diminished frequency

The key is to minimize the negative choices you make and increase the positive choices. So let's move on to discussing some positive choices you can make today.

The key to maintaining health is rooted in maintaining a high personal frequency.

Chapter 4

Essential Oils, Frequency & Better Health

Earlier, we revealed that simply inhaling an authentic therapeutic grade essential oil took a man's frequency from 52MHz (post coffee drinking) to 66Hz in just 21 seconds. Upon reading that you may have wondered (even questioned or disbelieved), "How the heck did that happen?" The answer is that essential oils are high in frequency.

Clinical research shows essential oils have the highest frequency of any natural substance known to man.[28] The oil with the lowest frequency is basil, which measures 52MHz. Many essential oils have frequencies that are over

---

Clinical research shows essential oils have the highest frequency of any natural substance known to man.

---

[28] http://www.bodymindconnection.com/health-pages/essential-oil.html

100MHz. The two highest are Australian blue cypress, with the incredible frequency of 522MHz and rose, with an impressive 320MHz. (Fascinating that one of the highest frequency oils comes from a flower symbolizing love).

What is particularly interesting about essential oils and their relationship to frequency is that research conducted at Weber State University, in Ogden, Utah . . . ."indicates that most viruses, fungi, and bacteria cannot live in the presence of most essential oils, especially those high in phenol, carvacrol, thymol, and terpenes. . . (and) a vast body of anecdotal evidence (testimonials) suggests that those who use essential oils are less likely to contract infectious diseases."[29]

When you stop and think about the effectiveness of essential oils in disease prevention it makes sense. If disease states begin at 58MHz, by using something that would boost ones' frequency higher than 58MHz should help to maintain good health.

The following are tables showing the frequencies of Young Living Essential Oil:[30]

Single essential oils

Angelica	85 MHz
Basil	52 MHz

---

[29] Essential Oil Desk Reference, 2011, Life Science Publishers, 5th edition, p. 1.10

[30] Essential Oil Desk Reference, 2011, Life Science Publishers, 5th edition, p. 4.71

Frankincense	147 MHz
Galbanum	56 MHz
German Chamomile	105 MHz
Helichrysum	181 MHz
Idaho Tansy	105 MHz
Juniper	98 MHz
Lavender	118 MHz
Melissa (lemon balm)	102 MHz
Myrrh	105 MHz
Peppermint	78 MHz
Ravinsara	134 MHz
Rose	320 MHz
Sandalwood	96 MHz
Blue Cypress	522 MHz

Essential oil blends

Abundance	78 MHz
Acceptance	102 MHz
Aroma Life	84 MHz
Aroma Siez	64 MHz
Awaken	89 MHz
Brain Power	78 MHz
Christmas Spirit	104 MHz
Citrus Fresh	90 MHz
Clarity	101 MHz
Di-Gize	102 MHz
Dragon Time	72 MHz
Dream Catcher	98 MHz
EndoFlex	138 MHz
En-R-Gee	106 MHz
Envision	90 MHz

Exodus II	180 MHz
Forgiveness	192 MHz
Gathering	99 MHz
Gentle Baby	152 MHz
Grounding	140 MHz
Harmony	101 MHz
Hope	98 MHz
Humility	88 MHz
ImmuPower	89 MHz
Inner Child	98 MHz
Inspiration	141 MHz
Into the Future	88 MHz
Joy	188 MHz
Juva Flex	82 MHz
Live w/ Passion	89 MHz
Magnify Your Purpose	99 MHz
Melrose	48 MHz
Mister	147 MHz
Motivation	103 MHz
M-Grain	72 MHz
PanAway	112 MHz
Peace & Calming	105 MHz
Present Time	98 MHz
Purification	46 MHz
Raven	70 MHz
R.C.	75 MHz
Release	102 MHz
Relieve It	56 MHz
Sacred Mt.	176 MHz
SARA	102 MHz
Sensation	88 MHz

Surrender	98 MHz
Thieves	150 MHz
3 Wise Men	72 MHz
Trauma Life	92 MHz
Valor	47 MHz
White Angelica	89 MHz

Some interesting history on frequency

In the early 1920's, Royal Raymond Rife, M.D, developed a device to treat and cure cancer. It was officially called a Beam Ray machine, now referred to as the Rife Generator, and it generated frequencies with electromagnetic energy. By using certain frequencies he could alter a cancer cell or virus. He also believed that frequency therapy could prevent the development of all disease.

It is documented in various places, some of which are now on the Internet, that in 1934 the University of Southern California appointed a team of doctors and pathologists to test the device on terminally ill cancer patients. After three months doctors determined that fourteen of the patients were cured, and with the other two having additional, adjusted treatments, they also ultimately were cured.

Supposedly Dr. Rife received honors and accolades from the most respected doctors and scientists. However, by the end of the 1930's he was being criticized. His work discredited and he escaped to Mexico while others from his research team were brought to trial and sentenced to prison terms.

Although it is unclear as to exactly why all this happened, many believe that the medical establishment, particularly the pharmaceutical giants, were so threatened by the potential development of a cure for disease that they used their influence and power to discredit Rife. Whether that is true or not doesn't really matter. What is important is that in the 1990's the Rife Generator technology was rediscovered and has spawned additional, more advanced health and wellness devices that integrate frequency functions.

In fact, for those interested there is an entire field of science called Quantum Physics, which delves very deeply into the understanding of energetics (and frequency) as it relates to health. It is a very "deep" and complex subject, and is not for the faint of heart. And yes, the medical establishment and pharmaceutical companies still work hard to discredit the information, but with the power of the Internet more and more people are beginning to explore and appreciate the magnitude of this growing research.

Frequency, oils, & your body

If you have a scientific mind you may still be asking yourself, "But exactly how is it that an increase in frequency ends up having a positive impact on ones' health?" The layman's answer is simply what we have been discussing; disease cannot survive when your frequency (energy) is high enough—i.e. above 58MHz.

The logic that follows is that by using essential oils that have frequencies higher than 58MHz, you can positively impact your own frequency. For those that have an understanding of physics, that explanation is too simple. These individuals believe that the concept of amplitude must also be taken into consideration when trying to explain why essential oils have such incredible, medicinal effects.

We promised you we wouldn't get too technical so let's try to keep this simple. Evelyn Vincent, on her Blog, "The Very Essence", made a very informative entry regarding this subject.[31] To paraphrase the long post, she defined amplitude as the maximum displacement (of a wave) during one period of oscillation. That meant nothing to us until she showed a picture!

If you look at the figure below you will see a wavy line, which is representative of a wave. Amplitude, which is measured vertically, would be the peaks and valleys. Frequency, which is measured horizontally, is measured in length from left to right. A higher frequency will produce a longer wave and greater amplitude will produce higher peaks and valleys.

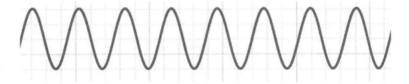

---

[31] http://aromatherapy4u.wordpress.com/2008/09/22/can-you-raise-your-frequency-with-essential-oils/

This is depicted best with the screen shot below, which is a visual representation of voice that was recorded using editing software. The first third of the wave is a whisper, the middle is normal volume, and the final third is yelling. Look at the huge changes in the amplitude.

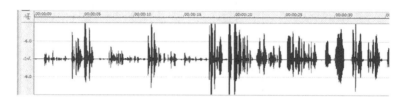

Vincent, through much explanation and visual support, explains how the amplitude of an oils' frequency is what changes the dominant frequency. It's a bit technical, but the ultimate effect is a change to the body's frequency.

One final interesting point is that oils actually affect different parts of the body because body parts have different frequencies (see chart). Therefore, different oils will naturally resonate with different body parts. Although this is a very primitive explanation of an incredibly complex subject, it helps to explain the seemingly mysterious impact therapeutic grade essential oils have and why so many people around the world tell seemingly miraculous stories of healing. Below is a short list of common organs and their frequencies:

Thyroid and Parathyroid glands are 62-68 MHz
Thymus Gland is 65-68 MHz
Heart is 67-70 MHz
Lungs are 58-65 MHz

Liver is 55-60 MHz
Pancreas is 60-80 MHz
Stomach is 58-65 MHz
Ascending Colon is 58-60 MHz
Descending Colon is 58-63 MHz[32]

---

[32] http://www.heavenscentoils.net/frequency_of_essential_oils.htm

Chapter 5

Medical Research on Essential Oils

Many people are surprised to learn that there is a large body of scientific research on essential oils. In fact, in the National Library of Medicine, which is the largest medical library in the world, essential oils are represented in almost 10,000 studies.[33] In *Scent to Heal and Anoint*, the author lists a number of studies.[34]

- A study at Wythenshawe Hospital in Manchester, England found that a vaporizer diffusing a blend of East Indian lemongrass (cymbopogan flexuosus), and sweet-scented geranium (Pelargonium graveolens) into the air effectively reduced airborne bacteria, including methicillin-resistant Staphylococcus aureus (known commonly as MRSA), by 89% when operated for 15 hours.

---

[33] Essential Oil Desk Reference, 2011, Life Science Publishers, 5th edition, p. 1.27

[34] Direct quotes, Scent to Heal and Anoint, Linda Smith, 2011, 6th edition, p. 52-54

- 2001. A clinical trial of 224 human subjects infected with MRSA found that tea-tree preparation was effective in treating MRSA. They found that almost as many patients receiving treatment with the tea tree oil products were free of MRSA (41%) as were patients receiving the control, a standard treatment of the antibiotic mupirocin, chlorhexidine gluconate, and silver sulfadiazine (49%). While the standard antibiotic treatment was more effective in killing MRSA in the nasal region, the tea tree cream and body wash were better at clearing MRSA from the skin and wounds. Another study reported that aerosolized tea tree oil reduced hospital-acquired infections.

- Much more extensive than the body of existing human studies is the collection of *in vitro* research. Cinnamon, thyme, lemon, lemon balm, lemongrass, sage, clary sage, and eucalyptus oils have been found to be active against several bacterial strains, such as MRSA, S. aureus, E. Coli, S. epidermidis, Candida krusei, S. pneumonia, Haemophilus influenza, and Moraxella catarrhalis.

- The most powerful antifungal essential oils: Cinnamon bark, cassia, cinnamon leaf, clove, bay laurel, basil, lemongrass, rose, cumin, geranium and thyme. The essential oils of cinnamon, clove, lemongrass, geranium and thyme were equal or superior to the powerful anti-fungal drug, Hexaconazole.

- In 1987, one of the most comprehensive studies conducted by scientists in Scotland identified the most powerful antibacterial essential oils to be thyme, cinnamon, clove and geranium. Cinnamon, thyme and clove essential oils killed 92% of 25 different gram negative and positive bacterial strains in another research study published in the International Journal of Food Microbiology.

- Essential oils even when diluted, kill bacteria that antibiotics do NOT. Melaleuca, lavender, peppermint and thyme essential oils showed the strongest killing power against MRSA (methicillin-resistant Staphylococcus aureus) and VRE (vancomycin-resistent Enterococcus faecium).

There are also many studies done on the effect of essential oils and cancer treatment. Dr. H.K. Lin, assistant professor at the Oklahoma University College of Medicine, has been conducting research on the use of frankincense with bladder cancer. Lin notes, *". . . lab testing found an extract of the Somali frankincense tree Boswellia carteri can kill off bladder cancer cells, while leaving normal cells*

There are also many studies done on the effect of essential oils and cancer treatment.

---

intact. "[35] His research has been published in the journal BioMed Central, which focuses on complimentary and alternative medicines.

Dr. Mahmoud Suhail, an Iraqi pediatrician, in collaboration with an international team, has discovered that frankincense seems to have an extraordinary effect on cancer cells. He explains, "Essentially, it (frankincense) reprograms the nucleus so that it no longer believes it's a cancer cell, and the surrounding cell is then destroyed . . . like reformatting a computer."[36]

Dr. Suhail and Dr. Lin collaborate together on their research. Suhail sends Lin a variety of frankincense samples from different regions using different extraction methods. Lin, in turn uses them in his testing on pancreatic, bladder, and breast cancer cells. Suhail is very optimistic about the results. He states, "We're pretty sure that it (frankincense) will be more helpful to cancer patients than most drugs currently available. And personally, I think that it will be more helpful to cancer patients than all current anti-cancer drugs. It's a huge discovery. Nobody has done this before – changed the DNA of cancer cells. It could be as revolutionary as the discovery of penicillin."[37]

These are just a few of the highlights regarding essential oil research. More and more countries, universities, scientists, and doctors are beginning to at least recognize that nature's

[35] http://newsok.com/article/3354293
[36] http://www.geographical.co.uk/Magazine/Oman_-_Mar_11.html
[37] http://www.geographical.co.uk/Magazine/Oman_-_Mar_11.html

first medicines—essential oils and herbs—can offer significant contributions to health practitioners and their patients and, in some instances, be more effective without the side effects of pharmacology.

As recently as April of 2012, the *Health & Wellness* section of the *Wall Street Journal* had a half-page article featuring the newest advancements of herbs as enhancers in chemotherapy treatments.[38] Today, with works being published in medical journals and being validated in clinical trials his research is getting the interest and respect for which he had hoped.

---

[38] "Chinese Medicine Goes Under the Microscope, The Wall Street Journal, Tuesday, April 3, 2012, p. D4

Chapter 6

Understanding Essential Oils

Now that we have some understanding of the power of essential oils, perhaps it's time to discuss what they are. The name actually generates a lot of confusion. Unlike vegetable oils that are greasy, essential oils are lipid soluble (can penetrate cell membranes). They are the "aromatic, volatile liquid that is within many shrubs, flowers, trees, roots, bushes and seeds."[39] That liquid—i.e. the oil—is the life-force of the plant, carrying vital nutrients that protect it from infections and diseases.

A good way to think of it is that essential oil is to the plant what blood is to humans. Basically, it is a transport mechanism that carries all of the vital elements that help to keep it alive and healthy. If you cut yourself, you bleed. If you tear or

A good way to think of it is that essential oil is to the plant what blood is to humans.

[39] Essential Oil Desk Reference, 2011, Life Science Publishers, 5th edition, p. 1.3

snip a plant, it "bleeds." In both those processes, a substance
is rushed to the location of the cut to help it fight off infection,
seal off the bleeding, and carry oxygen for repair.

Because essential oils flow throughout an entire plant, most
are extracted through steam distillation. After the plants
are harvested, they are placed in what could be described
as a huge cooker. A lid is placed on top of the container
and then steam is forced through it. When the steam comes
in contact with the plant material, it "ruptures the plant's
oil-bearing sacs and cavities and frees the oil which then
evaporates into the steam. The steam and vaporized oil
is passed out of the chamber and through a coiled tube
surrounded by cold water that condenses the steam and oil
into a liquid. It is then collected into another chamber."[40]

Although it sounds simple enough, the process is very delicate.
Every essential oil has different properties and a given
temperature will affect each oil uniquely. If the temperature is
too high, some of the valuable properties can be lost; keep the
temperature too low and some might not be extracted.

In a later section we will discuss the importance of the quality
of essential oils and how you can be certain to purchase a
brand that offers the purest, most therapeutic quality.

Man's first medicine

Many people do not realize that pharmacology, as we know
it today has its roots in plants. Most medicines have an

---

[40] <u>Scent to Heal and Anoint</u>, Linda Smith, 2011, 6th edition, p. 46

active ingredient that simulates one or more constituents of a plant. One of the most common would be any type of topical pain cream, which utilizes the properties of menthol. Menthol is the key constituent in peppermint oil, accounting for up to 44% of the extracted material. The menthol in the products you buy at the pharmacy is almost always chemically reproduced. Furthermore, the cream usually has a petrochemical base.

What this means is that you smell the menthol, your skin gets the same tingly sensation as if it were nature's menthol, but the effects on your body are *not* the same as they would be if peppermint oil had been used.

Another more extreme example is the use of WD-40 on human body parts to lubricate their joints and reduce pain. (Yes, some people do this and If you don't believe me then just Google "WD-40 for joint relief" and see the evidence!) It may accomplish the desired outcome but the side effects on the liver are severe. You don't want to use drugs for relief of one issue when it will create another one.

References to the use of essential oils can be traced to Egyptian papyrus manuscripts as far back as 2800 B.C. There are many hieroglyphics on the walls of Egyptian temples that depict the use of oils and their recipes. In fact,

---

Most medicines have an active ingredient that simulates one or more constituents of a plant.

---

the Ebers Papyrus, an Egyptian medical scroll dated 1550 B.C., outlines 877 different prescriptions using essential oils.[41]

All living things, including essential oils, are made up of carbon, hydrogen, and oxygen compounds. These compounds fall into two basic groups: hydrocarbons and oxygenated compounds.[42]

"In 1922, when King Tutankhamen's tomb was opened, some 50 alabaster jars designed to hold 350 liters of oils were discovered."[43]

The bible also has hundreds of references to essential oils and scents, including the gifts brought to Jesus upon his birth, which included frankincense and myrrh. The book *Healing Oils, Healing Hands,* gives a wonderful account of how oils were used during the time of Christ and why the people of that time placed a higher value than gold on certain oils because of their medicinal properties.

References to the use of essential oils can be traced to Egyptian papyrus manuscripts as far back as 2800 B.C.

---

[41] http://www.crystalinks.com/egyptmedicine.html
[42] Scent to Heal and Anoint, Linda Smith, 2011, 6th edition, p. 47
[43] Essential Oil Desk Reference, 2011, Life Science Publishers, 5th edition, p. 1.6

History also tells us that the Greeks used essential oils. In the temples of Aesculapius and Aphrodite, there were recipes for a number of medicinal oils inscribed on marble tablets. Hippocrates, the famous Greek scholar, is quoted as saying: "The way to health is to have an aromatic bath and scented massage every day".[44] The skeptic might note that Hippocrates didn't use the exact words "essential oils" in this statement but, put in the context of what we know of during his time, most believe he was referring to essential oils.

Many other countries like India and China have long since used aromatics, herbs, and essential oils as well as have the native Indians in the U.S. and Canada and the Aborigines in Australia and New Zealand. Throughout time and cultures, people have used these gifts of nature to treat physical conditions as well as emotional and spiritual support.

You may be wondering, "If people have been using essential oils and aromatics for thousands of years for medicinal purposes, why have I never heard of it?" That's a valid question and one we can only answer by way of logical reasoning.

First, because essential oils were so revered and valuable, it was usually the very wealthy who had access to them. Second, because of their unavailability, common people turned to plants and dried herbs. It was commonplace for every household to have an herb garden.

---

[44] Scent to Heal and Anoint, Linda Smith, 2011, 6th edition, p. 25

If you are old enough, you may remember your grandmother having one and making you a fresh cup of peppermint tea when you had a stomach ache. However, like sewing, baking, preserving, and other once-common daily activities, western society sped up and very few people today have any kind of garden—never mind growing their own herbs! The age old process of handing down life skills and knowledge from one generation to the next has, unfortunately deteriorated.

Finally, advancements in science and the ability to chemically manufacture medicines made it economically advantageous to produce large amounts of products at a fraction of the cost (and in a lot less time) than with plants. This also created the commercial motivation for manufacturers and whole industries to actively discredit competitors who offer alternatives, like essential oils.

There may be other reasons, but what we know is history tells us that people used herbs and essential oils for a very long time but they fell out of everyday use.

Fortunately, because of a very unfortunate accident involving Rene-Maurice Gattefosse, Ph.D., a French cosmetic chemist, they were reintroduced in the early

---

What we know is history tells us that people used herbs and essential oils for a very long time but they fell out of everyday use.

1900's. As the story is told, Dr. Gattefosse was working in a lab when an explosion occurred, and his hands were engulfed in flames. After the flames were extinguished he put his hands into a bucket of lavender thinking it was water. Miraculously his hands healed and, being a scientist, he began studying the chemistry of essential oils, later publishing a book in 1937 entitled *Aromatherapy.*

Dr. Gatttefosse then shared his work with a medical colleague, Dr. Jean Valnet, from Paris. Valnet served as a doctor in World War II and, when he ran out of antibiotics he began using essential oils on patients with battlefield injuries and had positive results.[45]

The basic chemistry of essential oils

Essential oils are truly amazing substances. Each essential oil is a complex structure of hundreds of different chemicals. "A single essential oil may contain anywhere from 80-300 or more different chemical constituents."[46] In the case of Clary Sage there are up to 900! Essential oils, like all living things, are made up of compounds that are composed of carbon, hydrogen, and oxygen, sulfur, and nitrogen.

There are 13 categories of essential oil constituents: Alkanes, phenols, terpenes, alcohols, ethers, aldehydes,

---

[45] Essential Oil Desk Reference, 2011, Life Science Publishers, 5th edition, p. 1.9
[46] Essential Oil Desk Reference, 2011, Life Science Publishers, 5th edition, p. 1.4

ketones, carboxylic acids, esters, oxides, lactones, coumarins, and furanoids. Each constituent has a different purpose to the plant and works in synergy for the survival of the plant species.

Every essential oil has elements of one or more of these constituents, and it is that unique combination that gives it a specific application for medicinal purposes. Esters are calming, relaxing, and can be anti-fungal and antispasmodic. Phenols are anti-bacterial, anti-infectious, and antiseptic. Sesquiterpenes are anti-bacterial, anti-inflammatory, antiseptic, and sedative. Ketones have decongestant and analgesic benefits. It is the complexity of essential oils that makes them so powerful and prevents duplication in a laboratory setting.

The Chemistry of Essential Oils Made Simple by David Stewart, Ph.D., D.N.M, is a wonderful, 800-plus-page resource that goes into great detail how essential oils work. If you don't like chemistry, the book may initially scare you, but if you take it in bits and pieces and use it as more of a reference, your understanding of the subject will be enriched. For those needing the more scientific explanation of how oils work, please take the time to read it.

For others who just want to know why essential oils work the answer is simple. Because essential oils are the closest thing in chemical makeup to human blood known to man, they become transport mechanisms for the constituents that they carry. Once introduced into your cells they have an affect on the body.

For example, essential oils can stimulate the secretion of antibodies, neurotransmitters, endorphins, hormones, and enzymes. They can also increase the uptake of oxygen, and can enhance circulation and immune function. Most importantly, "because of their complexity, essential oils do not disturb the body's natural balance or homeostasis: if one constituent exerts too strong an effect, another constituent may block or counteract it. Synthetic chemicals, in contrast, usually have one action and often disrupt the body's homeostasis."[47]

Another interesting aspect about essential oils is their powerful immunity. As we have seen in recent years, certain viruses and bacteria create a resistance to antibiotics and other drugs. Because of the complexity of essential oils, combined with the fact that every harvest of oil is slightly different due to growing conditions (therefore a different chemical makeup every time), resistance is not an issue.

Because essential oils are the closest thing in chemical makeup to human blood known to man, they become transport mechanisms for the constituents that they carry. Once introduced into your cells they have an affect on the body.

---

[47] Essential Oil Desk Reference, 2011, Life Science Publishers, 5th edition, p. 1.19

We have intentionally covered just a few of the basics on the chemistry and history of essential oils. We hope that these few bits of information are enough to give you an appreciation for essential oils and, more importantly, a desire to begin using them.

Chapter 7

Learning How to Use Essential Oils

Once the decision to purchase and use essential oils is made, the next logical step is learning how to use them. The first kit I purchased from Young Living was the Raindrop Kit. The oil combo aims to help people with back issues (as well as other applications). I was so excited to get my box. I quickly took out all the little bottles, opened each one to give them a smell, and then realized I had no clue exactly what to do with them! Sure, I figured I should be putting them on my back (and the instructions told me the order I should follow), but lots of questions ran through my mind.

"Can I put them all on at once? Could there be any negative interactions with this many oils on my body in such a short period of time? Do I need to wash my hands in between applications of each oil?" These were just a few of the many questions I would ultimately have about using the oils. Perhaps, these types of questions have already crossed your mind.

There are several things that add to the mystique and confusion about the use of essential oils. First, because most governments do not recognize essential oils for therapeutic purposes their production and manufacturing falls under the category of perfume. As a result, you don't find instructions for therapeutic purposes on the bottle. In fact, most will always say, "For topical or aromatic use only" because laws require this labeling due to their classification.

Also, most people have limited or no exposure to essential oils. Some may see them in a health food store or located near incense products and assume their only use is casual aromatic enjoyment. Others may have had essential oils applied for a massage and believe they are used for sore muscles. Still others could have been introduced to oils from a naturopath who utilizes them, but these would be very small numbers.

Next, because the art of using essential oils had been lost for so many centuries, most people have no experience with them except for aromatic purposes. In fact, if you put a bottle of peppermint, lavender, or wintergreen and a bottle of Ibuprofen in the medicine cabinet of the average American or Australian, 9.9 times out of 10 they would grab the Ibuprofen if they had a headache.

The lack of knowledge and education about oils and the familiarity with using prescription and over-the-counter drugs as "the norm" means that people are more comfortable with grabbing pills—even combining several pills (like allergy medications) without thinking twice! How ironic.

An overview of how to use essential oils

As your knowledge of essential oils increases, so will your comfort level as it relates to exploring different ways to use them. But before you can run, you must walk, so let's quickly review the three most common ways in which you will use essential oils everyday:

- Inhalation
- Topical application
- Internal consumption.

1. Inhalation

The most common and easily accepted way to use essential oils is through inhalation. Although humans don't have near the number of olfactory glands as most animals, we are still very much influenced by smell. Think back to your childhood and ask yourself, "What was your most favorite aroma coming from your mother's kitchen?" Maybe it was fresh chocolate chip cookies, or perhaps the simmering of spaghetti sauce. Whatever it was, you have created a very strong association to that scent and it can evoke positive feelings just by recalling it in your mind!

People are more comfortable with grabbing pills—even combining several pills (like allergy medications) without thinking twice! How ironic.

The same holds true for scents with negative associations. If a person had a bad experience at a doctor's office or hospital he or she will get nauseous when they return to an environment that has those same odors.

A mutual friend of ours was a young boy when his mother wanted to have a family portrait painted. This involved a long, weekly car ride to the artist's studio. Because the young boy was prone to car sickness he would arrive at the artist's studio nauseous. At the outer entrance were many holly trees, which have a very strong fragrance. To this day—some 40+ years later—he feels sick at the sight of holly trees, even just the picture of a holly tree on a Christmas card evokes the feeling!

The bottom line is, our sense of smell has a powerful impact on our feelings and on certain body reactions.

Without getting into any serious discussion of anatomy, let's outline the basics of how inhaling essential oils works. The aroma from the oil is picked up in your nasal cavity and the receptor sites are triggered; this is your initial smell process. This in turn triggers the neurons from your olfactory senses, and the molecules from the oil are converted to an electrical impulse and are carried through the olfactory nerve into the amygdula (where

---

Our sense of smell has a powerful impact on our feelings and on certain body reactions.

---

emotions are stored), and the pineal and pituitary regions of the brain, which is referred to as the limbic region. The smell sensory cortex at the base of the brain stem records all activity in the limbic region. Now you have a memory of that smell.

Although it is smell that we have the most vivid recall of, it is the impact that the molecules have on the body itself that are giving the greatest therapeutic benefits.

As was discussed earlier in the Basic Chemistry section, the increase in oxygen by inhaling the essential oils triggers activity in the pineal and pituitary glands to produce hormones like Melatonin, HGH, FSH, and LH, which in turn can positively impact the immune system. This is just one aspect of how the inhalation of oils impacts the body.

The limbic system is connected to the parts of the brain that control heart rate, blood pressure, breathing, memory, stress levels, and hormone balance, which is why oils have both physiological and psychological effects on the body.[48] Although that may be too simple of an explanation for the more scientific readers or a too technical explanation for the layperson, the only thing you really need to understand is that inhaling essential oils is a good thing—physically, emotionally and even spiritually.

---

[48] Essential Oil Desk Reference, 2011, v5.0, p. 1.22

Ways to inhale

New users of essential oils often ask, "What is the best way to use the oils?" The response from seasoned "oilers" is simple—anyway! Knowing that you probably want a little more direction than that, here are five common ways in which you can inhale essential oils.

- **Diffuse**. With this method essential oils are sent into the air by one of several mechanical devices. Diffusers will quickly fill up a room with the wonderful fragrance of your choice and allow for continual inhalation of the aroma.

  As you would suspect, there are several different types of diffusers on the market each using different technology that claims to be the best. Although it is not our intention to recommend or endorse one particular brand over another, there is some evidence that ultrasonic diffusers are superior in their effect because they deliver micron-sized droplets of water into the air using high frequency sound without heat. (Therefore, you only have a small device that has a water-holding tank and an ionizer.)

  You place several drops of oil into the reservoir and the ionization causes the vapors to form and be released into the air, which has two benefits. First, there is no damage to the oil, which can happen when oils are heated. Many people make the mistake of using essential oil burners, which not only damage the oil but rob the air of oxygen and add sulfur! Second, the patterns of movement created from the sonic waves in the ionization process help to deliver more essential oil into the air, which means more oils into your nasal passages and a better physiological result.

A second type of diffuser that has been around for years is a nebulizer. This device works by attaching the bottle of essential oil onto a mechanism that holds water and has an air pump attached to it. The suction from the air pump pulls oil into the small water reservoir and then pushes it out into the room. Advocates of the newer ionic diffusers believe that this process can damage the oils and diminish their effectiveness.

Although only a scientist can settle that debate, I personally prefer the ionic diffuser for different reasons. For instance, I find the misting action of the diffuser very calming and most ionic diffusers have some kind of lighting that can also be very soothing—kind of like a lava lamp (however, you can turn off the lights for sleeping). Also, I find it more convenient to change aromas by simply putting a few drops of different oil in a new basin of water rather than having to fiddle with unscrewing bottles and locating the cap.

You can go online and find many, many different brands and models of diffusers with as many different price ranges. Certainly there is something to say for the notion of "you get what you pay for", so bear this in mind when making a selection. If a diffuser available online is a lot less than most other similar brands, it might not have a long life. Our suggestion is to invest in a quality diffuser so you get the most benefits and value for money.

One final note about diffusing—the more you can diffuse, the better, because ALL essential oils help to bring oxygen to the brain. Alan and I are admittedly "oil-a-holics" and have three of the same diffusers. One in the bedroom where calming oils like Lavender or Peace and Calming are used as a sleep aid; one in the office with oils high in oxygen-rich sesquiterpines, like sandalwood, frankincense, or Brain Power; and, one in the home with a fresh scent like lemon, citrus fresh, Thieves Blend, or Purification.

We both also have travel diffusers, which use a simple fan mechanism. This type of diffuser makes it easy and very convenient to diffuse while in the car or a hotel room. These usually offer the option of a battery or an AC adapter. You may find yourself laughing but I can assure you our surroundings always smell good and uplift our spirits and those of the people who visit us!

- **Bottle or hands**. I began our inhalation discussion with diffusers because I believe they are the best way to consistently and conveniently inhale oils.

Obviously, , the easiest way to inhale oils is by simply opening a bottle and bringing it up to your nose, or by placing a few drops of oil into your hands, bringing them up to your face, and taking a few deep breaths.

Using the bottle is always effective when you want a 'hit' of oil but don't want the after effects of having it on your hands. Some men like this method, particularly when the oil has a flowery scent. If you only want a quick smell, you would immediately put the cap back on, while at other times you can simply leave the cap off and place the bottle near you. This certainly won't be as aromatic or saturating to the senses as a diffuser, but it is a nice option.

When using the 'hand-inhalation' method, one suggestion is that you lightly rub your hands together in a circular motion three times before cupping your hands to your face. The reasoning behind this is that it activates the molecules while distributing the oils across a larger portion of the palms. Of course, with this method you get the

---

The easiest way to inhale oils is by simply opening a bottle and bringing it up to your nose, or by placing a few drops of oil into your hands, bringing them up to your face, and taking a few deep breaths.

---

added benefit of topical application, which we will be talking about soon.

- **Steam**. Another wonderful way to enjoy the benefits of essential oils through inhalation is with steam. If you are fortunate enough to have access to a steam room, it is simple to add a few drops of essential oil and it will quickly fill it up with the wonderful aroma of your choice. If you have aches or pains, you can add an oil topically to the area that is causing you discomfort and then go into the steam room. One word of caution here is that some oils "heat up" on your body, and the steam room will magnify their effect. Therefore, always test a small amount of any oil before going into a steam room.

  If you are a big fan of steam like we are but don't have access to a professional steam room (or steam shower in your house), there are companies that make steam pods. These are small one and two person capsules that become self-enclosed steam pods that you sit in.

  Although it was a considerable investment, I use mine all the time and it is a place of respite for friends and family members who are dealing with congestion from coughs and colds. It can be put anywhere, it plugs into a regular electrical outlet and is self-contained, needing no external plumbing or drainage. It takes distilled water and has a small, thimble-like, removable reservoir to place a few drops of oil into. It can't be simpler! Also, my unit is now more than 10 years old and still running strong.

There are less expensive ways to enjoy the benefits of steam inhalation. You can add a few drops to a wet face cloth and place it over the top portion of the showerhead so in a hot shower the steam releases the oils without washing them out of the cloth. And, there is always "Mom's favorite" remedy for blocked sinuses, which is to boil a pot of water, put a couple of drops in and position your head over the steam with a towel acting like a tent over your head. I can vividly remember doing this as a child, but seem to remember something like Vicks Vapor Rub being put in the pot, which has some amounts of eucalyptus in it but also has petrochemicals so it is not recommended.

- **Vents and materials**. One final way that you can get some inhalation benefits from essential oils is by applying several drops onto vents. A vent could be anything from the fins of a heating or air conditioning system to the vents in your car. Whatever the source of vent, adding the oils topically to where air or steam passes will cause the aroma to be sent through the air in some capacity. One simply way to accomplish this is by placing several drops on a cotton ball and positioning it in front of the vent. An important note is that you never want to add essential oils into the water of a humidifier because it will float on top and not effectively be released into the air.

Finally, if for some reason none of these other methods are readily available to you, simply put a few drops of oil on a tissue, cotton ball, or other piece of cloth material and place it near you. This is a nice option of you are staying in someone else's home and are trying to be mindful of not sending too much scent into the air but still wanting the aromatic benefits that you desire.

2. Topically

Earlier, we outlined some very basic aspects of the chemistry of essential oils and how they work. You may remember that the essential oil extracted from plants is the closest substance to human blood known to man. Furthermore, because the lipid-soluble structure of essential oils is so similar to the makeup of human cell membranes, oils have the ability to penetrate the body and get into the

---

Because the lipid-soluble structure of essential oils is so similar to the makeup of human cell membranes, oils have the ability to penetrate the body and get into the tissue and blood system immediately.

---

tissue and blood system immediately.[49] This is why topical application of essential oils is so powerful.

One of the reasons most people don't initially think to apply oils topically is because of the word 'oil.' Let's face it, "oil" predisposes us to believe that an essential oil will feel and act in the same way any other oil would—thick and greasy, not easily absorbed, and needing soap or some kind of stronger detergent to remove residue.

Therefore, most people are amazed to find that within a minute or two of putting an essential oil on their body, it is completely absorbed, leaving no trace of application. Also, if you get an essential oil on clothing it usually comes out in the wash without needing any special treatment.

Be smart!

Although therapeutic grade essential oils are safe, they are also powerful. In particular, if you have used a lot of personal care products that are high in petrochemicals (see earlier section regarding what impacts your health), you may have some initial sensitivity. Therefore, it is always smart to test a drop or two on your body before using larger amounts, gradually work up in amounts, and even dilute oils when starting use.

---

[49] Essential Oil Desk Reference, 2011, v5.0, p.1.18

Later in this book we have an entire section dedicated to the safety precautions when using and storing essential oils. Please read this entire section before beginning to enjoy your oils.

Where to apply oils

The only two places that you absolutely never want to come in contact with any oil are the eyes and inside the ears.[50] Other than those areas, it is possible to apply oils to any part of the body. That being said, there are several methodologies that are common when it comes to application choices. Let's review them here.

- **On a desired area**. Many people are introduced to essential oils because of a specific issue they are having, and someone recommends they try an oil either in lieu of a "traditional" treatment, or because a pharmaceutical choice didn't work or had bad side effects. In my case, I was having back pain even though I was taking 4-6 ibuprofens daily. Therefore, it made sense that I put the oils directly onto the area where I was having pain. If you have knee pain, put your oils of choice on the knee; if you have a headache, put them directly on the area from which your headache is being generated—i.e. temples, back of neck, etc.

---

[50] For an ear infection you can a small amount of essential oil on a small piece of cotton ball and place just inside your ear entrance.

The same concept holds true even when the issue isn't pain. For example, there are many skin issues that essential oils can help with. If you had a burn, you could apply lavender directly (or a spray product from Young Living called LavaDerm); if you wanted to reduce fine lines and wrinkles you could put one of several oils around the eye where smile lines develop (remember not to get the oil in your eye and some people may want to dilute the oil when using around the eye until they are accustomed to the process). Both these categories (pain and skin aid) are physical in nature, yet you still want to follow the same rules when using the oils for emotional support. So, if you were feeling blue you might place an uplifting oil or blend on your heart or the appropriate Chakra points, which is the name used for seven energy points of the body according to some eastern cultures. For a good overview and understanding of Chakras, go to:

www.spiritualnetwork.net/chakra/index.html

It may sound a bit ambiguous, but many of the choices you will make relating to where you apply certain oils will be intuitive in nature. That is, YOU will know where to put the oil on your body. For example, I love the oil blend called Magnify Your Purpose. There is no "instruction" on where to place it, but I have found that for me rubbing a small amount on my temples and under my nose has the greatest effect. However, you may find that another area works better for you.

By remembering that oils are working with <u>your</u> body—physically and emotionally—you begin to realize and appreciate that every essential oil has a unique impact for each individual. This is both the beauty and curse of essential oils—beauty because one oil can have many different uses and applications; curse because this variability does not always make people feel comfortable when beginning their journey with essential oils.

Always follow safety guidelines and use common sense, but know that in most cases putting any authentic therapeutic grade essential oil on the body is better than none.

Experiment with different oils for any one issue, and discover which ones resonate more with your body, similar to what you would do when trying to find your favorite nutritional foods or supplements. Keep good notes and soon enough you will have

---

By remembering that oils are working with <u>your</u> body—physically and emotionally—you begin to realize and appreciate that every essential oil has a unique impact for each individual.

---

your very own instruction manual for any issue that comes up in your life.

- **On the feet**. If you have had any exposure to reflexology, you know that it is the practice of applying pressure to the feet or hands, using thumb or finger techniques, with the goal of achieving physical changes in the body. The change happens because certain areas of the feet and hands represent zones or relate to specific areas of the body. For example, the tips of your big toes are connected to your brain; a certain point midway down the arch of your foot is connected to your adrenal glands; the curve along the inside ball of your foot relates to your spine.

  An individual trained in reflexology can look at a person's foot and, depending upon conditions that may be present—like calluses or bunions in particular areas of the foot—can identify a specific medical condition or imbalanced body function.

  For anyone not familiar with this practice, or other "non-traditional" therapies, it can seem a bit bizarre, but the practice of reflexology is documented in Archeological evidence dating back as early as 2330 B.C. in Egypt.

  A therapy similar to reflexology is called the Vita Flex Technique.

"Vita-Flex means 'vitality through the reflexes.' It is a specialized form of reflexive massage that uses rolling and releasing motions to activate reflex points on the feet, hands and various areas throughout the entire body. It is a tremendous tool that assists the body in healing itself, and is particularly effective in delivering the benefits of essential oils throughout the body. . . . it is based on a complete system of the internal workings of the body and the electrical circuitry inherent to the body."[51]

When using the Vita-Flex Technique on the feet in conjunction with essential oils, "an electrical charge is released that sends energy through the neuroelectrical pathways. This electrical charge follows the pathways of the nervous system to where there is a break in the electrical circuit, usually related to an energy block caused by toxins, damaged tissue, or loss of oxygen."

The biggest difference between reflexology and the Vita-Flex Technique is the hand technique. Reflexology uses constant pressure, where Vita-Flex uses a rolling and releasing motion. Although there are Vita-Flex charts for both the hands and feet, individuals who combine Vita-Flex with oils

---

[51] http://www.therealessentials.com/vitaflex.html

usually work with the feet. A simple Google search will provide you with a Vita-Flex Foot Chart.

- **On the ears**. There are three muscles that surround the outer ear, or auricular. Auricular therapy, developed by a French neurologist, is based on the idea that the auricular is a microsystem of the entire body and there are pressure points that can help to stimulate certain organs and emotions. One way to think of this would be acupuncture or acupressure of the ear, similar in concept to reflexology and Vita-Flex discussed above.

  D. Gary Young developed a technique called the Neuro Auricular Technique or NAT. This technique combines acupressure to the ear with authentic therapeutic grade essential oils. For those interested in using this technique, ear charts have been developed that identify pressure points for both emotional and physical issues. These diagrams can be found in the Essential Oil Desk Reference (EODR). A later chapter in this book will provide you with resources, including the contact information for the company that publishes the EODR.

- **On the spine**. You now know that the feet, hands and ears all have trigger points that are connected to and influence other functions and organs of the body and mind. It will come as no surprise then when we tell you that the same holds true for the spine. Of all the places of influence, the spine seems most obvious for this type of connection. Your entire nervous system runs through your spine. In fact, each vertebrae impacts specific glands or organs; there is a chart for this as well.

But beyond the connection to organs and bodily functions, there are many medical professionals who believe that viruses and bacteria lay dormant in the spine. This can cause inflammation—either local or systemic—which can result in spinal mis-alignment and ultimately a weakening of the body's immune system. Because of this and the fact that our entire nervous system runs through the spine, applying oils to this location makes sense.

One particular therapy using essential oils is called the Raindrop Technique. You may remember that my first introduction to essential oils involved the oils used in this technique. The big difference was that I only had the oils applied by Alan to my spine while bent over a chair; the actual Raindrop Technique is more like a massage, where a combination of essential oils, Vita-Flex, and specific oil application techniques are combined to deliver a wonderful experience that provides spinal health benefits.

"The Raindrop Technique uses high quality, authentic pure, organic, therapeutic grade essential oils which are dispensed like little drops of rain

from a height of about six inches above the
back, mixed with a variety of very light massage
techniques along the vertebrae and back muscles,
and Vita-Flex massage."[52]

- **In a bath**. As we have mentioned before, your skin
  is your largest organ and absorbs what is put on it
  topically. Adding essential oils to a nice, relaxing
  bath is a wonderful way to enjoy the oils topically
  and also aromatically while the warm water creates
  a vapor effect. Because water and oil do not mix, it
  is important that you put several drops of oils onto
  plain bath salts prior to adding them to the water to
  act as dispersing agents.

As you can see, there are many different ways in which you
can apply essential oils. There really is no "wrong" way to
apply oils, so enjoy experimenting and noticing what you
prefer.

Body-mind connection?

Most of us are familiar with the concept of the mind-body
connection, i.e., that your body will respond to the way you
think and feel. People who are obsessively fearful of getting
sick often have their biggest fears come true while someone
else who is legitimately sick thinks their way back to health.

---

[52] http://www.healingyourbody.net/index_files/Page17804.htm

If you believe in a mind body connection then you are probably open to the concept of a body-mind connection. Specifically, that feeding your body what it wants to be healthy can and will result in a better mental state. Let's face it, most people feel better when physically fit.

Essential oils work both of these "connections." They quickly impact the brain to make us feel better emotionally and they topically help us feel better physically. Each of these improved mental and physical states helps to support each other. For those who already use essential oils this makes perfect sense. For those yet to have such experiences simply be aware of the multi-dimensional impact essential oils will have on you.

3. Internal consumption

People who regularly use essential oils find that internal consumption offers the greatest benefits but it is also the most misunderstood and somewhat controversial practice. There are several reasons for this controversy. First, although regulated by the FDA, essential oils fall under the category of perfumes. This allows manufacturers have a tremendous leeway in their production standards because they are not being regulated as a medicine. For example, many oil manufacturers add synthetic chemicals to enhance the smell or increase the volume of material, thereby driving down costs. This is commonly referred to in essential oil literature as "adulterating oils."

Second, some manufacturers will add a vegetable oil, which is another way of reducing the per bottle cost while being able to still say 100% pure oil. Sure, it's all oil, but it's not pure, therapeutic grade essential oil! Either of these changes will reduce the effects of an oil, and ingesting an oil that has been adulterated may be harmful.

A third reason for controversy arises from the growing and harvesting processes. If the plants are not grown without pesticides, then those chemicals can be present in the plant itself, which means there can be small amounts in the final distilled product.

Finally, the distillation process dramatically influences the quality of the essential oil. Like vegetables that lose all their enzymes when overcooked, essential oils can lose their valuable medicinal properties if not distilled at a low temperature for the perfect amount of time. Because low-temperature distillation takes longer and is more costly, most manufacturers don't include it in their production process.

In fact, as we will discuss in a later section on choosing essential oils, you will learn that some brands simply buy oils from a variety of third party sources that have no quality control over their growing, distilling and manufacturing process. You do not want to be consuming oils that do not follow rigid quality control standards.

Another aspect that adds to the debate over internal use of essential oils is the fact that the FDA does not recognize oils for medicinal purposes. Those who oppose the internal use of oils use the "No FDA approval" as a way to scare consumers.

What most people don't know, however, is that both doctors and pharmacies in France prescribe essential oils internally for infections and diseases. Furthermore, there is a large naturopathic movement throughout the world that has discovered that using therapeutic grade essential oils internally can help with many conditions and diseases in lieu of prescription drugs. To see testimonials of individuals who successfully used essential oils internally, see the second half of this book.

The FDA does recognize many essential oils as Generally Regarded as Safe (GRAS). Other oils are recognized as a food additive (FA), which means they don't have a track record but are regarded as a safe food additive. All this information can be found on the FDA website; however, the list is all-inclusive, hence long and confusing. If you Google "Essential Oil GRAS list" you can find many websites that will provide you with a clear, comprehensive list of only the essential oils generally regarded as safe.

What most people don't know, however, is that both doctors and pharmacies in France prescribe essential oils internally for infections and diseases.

Adding essential oils like oregano, thyme or cinnamon to food dishes seems more commonplace. Most questions arise when consuming them for health benefits. There are actually many reasons why you might want to consume an essential oil.

For example, if you feel a cold approaching there are certain oils that can boost your immune system.

If you have a stomachache or an acute injury like a broken bone there are oils that can help provide relief.

Many people believe that internal use of certain oils provides greater benefits so long as the oils are pure. There are a variety of different ways in which you can consume oils.

- **Sub-lingual**. This is the Latin word for "beneath the tongue." There are advantages to sub-lingual administration. First, it can result in a faster absorption by the body because of the high number of capillaries underneath the tongue. Second, without having to be digested through the stomach and subjected to enzymes, heat, and acid, there is no degradation in strength. Remember that essential oils are sensitive to heat.

  For those choosing sub-lingual consumption of essential oils there is an added benefit; there is very limited taste underneath the tongue and a lower sensitivity. Since some essential oils have a strong taste this makes sub-lingual administration prefered over simply dropping them into the mouth.

Always test one drop of an oil under your tongue to determine your tolerance. If the sensation or flavor is too strong, immediately dilute with a vegetable oil, preferably a cold pressed olive oil, coconut oil or the Young Living V6 oil.

- **Gelatin capsule**. For those not wanting the sub-lingual option, another way to consume essential oils is with a vegetable based gelatin capsule. (That distinction is important because many gelatin capsules can be made of questionable materials.) Gelatin capsules are exactly that; a clear casing that allows you to make your own capsule of materials. Similar to going to the herb shop and making your own Echinacea capsules, you can make your own essential oil capsules. For strong or "hot" oils (like oregano), this is a nice alternative to the sub-lingual method. One word of advice is to make your capsules immediately before consumption. If you leave the liquid in the capsule for too long, it actually begins to melt and the oil will run out.

- **Added to liquids**. If you are opposed to sub-lingual use and have a hard time swallowing capsules, another option is to put the drops into a liquid drink. Putting oils that have a strong taste in beverages that are thicker seems to provide better masking; for example, any type of milk, (almond, rice, coconut, goat) or a smoothie of some sort. The goal with this approach is to use the smallest amount of liquid necessary to make drinking palatable.

Some oils actually help to enhance the flavor of beverages. For example:

o Adding Citrus Fresh (an oil blend), lemon, grapefruit, tangerine, orange, or peppermint to your water makes for a wonderful refreshment that is actually good for you! No need to purchase chemical-latent flavored waters anymore. BE CERTAIN to use either a glass, metal or BPA free bottle; remember that essential oils digest petrochemicals and therefore will break down plastic water bottles.

o A drop of orange into a smoothie enhances the fruit flavor without the added sugar.

o A drop of lavender into fresh-squeezed lemonade makes for a refreshing summer beverage.

o A drop of peppermint into peppermint tea greatly enhances the flavor. You can also add one drop of peppermint into a cup of hot cocoa for a fun, minty hot beverage during the cold months of winter.

o One friend of ours loves putting Thieves oil in his morning coffee. This turns his coffee into a chai like beverage.

• **Into food or when cooking**. If you need yet another option for oral consumption of oils, using food is simple. To completely mask the taste you can add drops to a spoonful of blue agave or honey. Kids and teens always prefer this choice. You can also put a drop or two on a piece of bread; the heartier the bread, the less you will taste the oil.

As was mentioned earlier, using essential oils in cooking is a wonderful way to enhance the flavors of your food. Basil, oregano, rosemary, and thyme are popular spices in most kitchens.

- Instead of using dried herbs, essential oils can add flavor with just one drop.

- Orange or lemon in frostings and baked goods is wonderful.

- Make your own, beautiful salad dressings and marinades without chemicals.

- If you like dipping bread into olive oil and spices, add one drop of essential oil and completely enhance the flavor. When having a party make different flavors for guests to try.

Using essential oils in cooking is a wonderful way to enhance the flavors of your food.

One final note about essential oils and cooking is when to add them. The general rule is to add them at the end of your cooking process to minimize their exposure to heat. Of course, with some things like cookie dough this is impossible.

Nasal irrigation

One additional category that is a hybrid of topical and ingestion is nasal irrigation. Just what it sounds like, this is the process of rinsing out the nasal cavity. Traditionally done to help relieve allergy, cold or flu symptoms there are several ways in which one can perform the process. One way is by using a neti pot, which is a small, ceramic pot that looks similar to a tea pot but the spout is designed to be inserted into one nostril; tip the head and gravity takes the liquid up one side and out the other. A nasal douche is the more commercial approach and this is simply a small spray bottle that you use to squirt into the nostrils one at a time. Both require a warm, salt water solution be added.

Essential oils are a wonderful addition to any type of nasal irrigation. One drop of any oil recommended for sinuses and you will add a power punch to the process. Of course, peppermint, eucalyptus and melaleuca will help to release and open sinus congestion while something like Thieves oil blend will help to kill bacteria and germs.

Whether it is internal, topical or through inhalation, you have many choices for using essential oils. Experiment and find the methods that suit your needs and personal taste.

What is most important is that you simply begin using essential oils in your life! The sooner you begin using oils, the sooner you will realize their effectiveness and the impact they can have on your well-being.

For a free User's Guide booklet go to http://keystoyoungliving. com/guide

Chapter 8

Essential Oil Safety & Selection

Now that you understand the basics of how to use essential oils, let's go over some safety guidelines.

- If you have any questions about personally using any essential oil product, consult a medical professional before beginning.

- If you are pregnant or nursing you should discuss the using of essential oil with your doctor.

- People with epilepsy or prone to convulsions should consult a health care professional before using essential oils.

- Read all label instructions before using.

- Never use any oil unless you are absolutely certain that it has not been diluted or adulterated, or if it contains a synthetic substitute. These items will be discussed at length in the next section, 'Choosing Essential Oils.'

- When using oils topically or internally, always go slowly. If your body has had a build up of toxins (as discussed in an earlier chapter), you may be sensitive to oils. This typically shows up as some kind of rash to the skin. Going slowly will ensure you avoid any undesired reactions while you become accustomed to the use of essential oils.

- Never put an essential oil directly into your eyes—it will cause irritation and will be very uncomfortable. If you should, by mistake, relax; you can stop the discomfort by simply placing a drop of olive oil (or other fatty oil) into your eye. You should instantly feel relief. Never try to dilute or wash an oil out with water, because water and oil do not mix and this will provide no relief.

- Never put any oil into your ear canal. (You can place a few drops of oil onto a cotton ball and place it in your ear canal.) You can use them on any portion of the outside of your ear. If you do get an essential oil into your ear, follow the same instructions as were given above regarding the eye. Place a drop near the ear canal and tilt your head until the oil has relieved any discomfort.

- Some oils, like oregano, cinnamon, and clove are considered 'hot'. This means that for some people they may cause minor skin irritation or sensitivity. A "heating up" on the skin's surface or redness is most common. Later in the book, for your convenience,

we have a list of oils that are considered 'hot.'
You can dilute these oils with a fatty oil prior to
applying, or if you begin to have sensitivity you can
then apply the oil calmative for immediate relief.

- Citrus oils (lemon, orange, tangerine, and
  grapefruit) are photosensitive. It is best to not use
  them topically if you plan on being out in the sun.

- Never mix an essential oil with another lotion
  or personal care product that contains synthetic
  substances. Most products you buy from a standard
  pharmacy or grocery store will fall into this category.

- Do not handle contact lenses right after your fingers
  have been in contact with any essential oil. This
  could result in irritation to the eye, and even small
  amounts of essential oil can damage lenses.

- Keep bottles closed at all times, or else they will
  evaporate!

- Keep the oils out of direct sunlight and high heat.

- Keep essential oils out of the reach of children.

If you did not download the free User's Guide to Essential
Oils that was mentioned at the end of the last chapter, you
may want to do that now. It provides an extensive, easy
to read application chart that makes recommendations

for each essential oil. Again, the link for that download is http://keystoyoungliving.com/guide

Mixing essential oils

One of the most common questions those new to essential oils have is, "Can I mix different oils together?" For example, if lemongrass is for muscle tension and clove is a high anti-oxidant, is there a benefit or a detriment to putting them together?

The simple answer is, "Yes, it is safe to mix pure essential oils together." The more complete answer is that there is actually an art and science to mixing. As we have mentioned earlier, essential oils are molecular, which means chemistry plays a role in mixing oils.

Specifically, each essential oil has a certain volatility, viscosity, and set of properties. When an oil has lighter and smaller molecules it will be thinner, more aromatic, and absorbed by the body faster. Heavier and larger molecules will mean an oil that is thicker, less aromatic, and slower absorbing. Therefore, if you are wanting a mixture of oils that works as quickly as possible (say on a physical ailment) you would choose oils that have smaller, lighter molecules. If you want a combination of oils that stays aromatic for a longer period of time you would need to combine just the right amount of lighter and heavier oils.

There may be times when you mix essential oils with what is called a "carrier" oil, which is any type of vegetable oil used for dilution. Dilution may be desired with stronger oils and is recommended on small children and small pets. If you are mixing essential oils with carrier oil, there are a couple of suggestions to follow. One, always use glass bottles with screw tops to ensure proper storage of your blend; and two, depending upon the amount of product you wish to make, fill your mixing bottle in a layering fashion, putting half the desired amount of carrier oil in first, adding the essential oil, and then topping off with carrier oil. This helps to mix the two together.

The good news is that just about any blend of essential oil you would want has already been mixed for you!

- Want the ideal mixture for improving your mood? Use Joy.
- Want the perfect mixture for pain relief? Use PanAway or Deep Relief.
- Need help relaxing and de-stressing? Use Peace and Calming.

As your experience with essential oils grows your willingness and confidence to make your own mixtures may grow. For the time being, feel good knowing that all the hard work has been done for you.

Choosing your essential oils

We have mentioned throughout this book the concern about ensuring you use only pure, therapeutic grade essential oils. Now that you have a more complete understanding of essential oil use and application, it is an appropriate time to delve deeper into this subject.

After the discussion on the effect toxins are having on your body and how cellular vitality impacts overall health, it is clear that for good health we only want to be using the best possible essential oils we can find. Unfortunately, there are a variety different grades of essential oils, and poor regulation and packaging laws make it simple for manufacturers to hide the ingredients of their product. Remember, essential oils fall under perfume standards as it relates to FDA regulation. Here are several different grades of essential oils:

- Grade A oils are pure authentic therapeutic quality. They usually are made from organically grown plants distilled at lower temperatures using steam distillation. In order to achieve therapeutic grade classification, each essential oil must achieve the designation naturally, without excess manipulation and refinement, and must meet specific criteria in four key areas: Plants, Preparation, Purity, and Potency. We will return to this discussion when we discuss the Seed to Seal® process.

It is clear that for good health we only want to be using the best possible essential oils we can find.

- Grade B oils are food grade. These may contain synthetics, pesticides, fertilizers, extenders, or filler oils, all of which cause adulteration.

- Grade C oils are perfume grade and may contain the same type of adulterating chemicals as food grade oils. They usually contain solvents, which are used to create more products with a small amount of actual oil. Solvents are toxic and can be cancerous.

You only want to use pure, therapeutic grade essential oils. Deciding that is easy; knowing which oils are actually pure isn't so simple. In fact, if you were to go down to your local health food store, the bottles of essential oils they have on their shelves will look nice, the product might smell nice, AND the bottle might say, "100% pure essential oil". It might even say "100% pure therapeutic essential oil". Unfortunately, no matter what it says, there is a good chance that it is not pure, not therapeutic, and not something you would want to inhale, put on your body, nor ingest.

Unless you know the exact planting, growing, harvesting, distillation, and bottling process of a particular essential oil, you don't want to risk using it for all the reasons we have

---

Unless you know the exact planting, growing, harvesting, distillation, and bottling process of a particular essential oil, you don't want to risk using it for all the reasons we have already stated.

---

already stated. Most essential oil products are bottled by a company that had nothing to do with the planting, growing, harvesting, or distillation. There is, however, one company that we know of that meticulously manages the entire process, ensuring consumers pure, therapeutic grade essential oils. It is called Young Living.

From Seed to Seal™

Young Living is the world leader in essential oils. D. Gary Young, ND, (naturopathic doctor) the founder, is committed to ensuring every single essential oil they bottle is therapeutic grade. Young Living is the only company in the world to develop the Seed to Sealä process, of which there are five steps:

1. <u>Seed</u>. Select seeds that are of the highest quality and that will produce the best result. Species certification involves scientific research, field study, university documentation, and on-site planting certification.

2. <u>Cultivate</u>. Soil preparation, proper irrigation, responsible weed and pest control, and wild-craft harvesting ensure the highest standards. Most importantly, plants need to be grown on uncontaminated soil that is free of fertilizers, pesticides and other chemicals used in most farming today. Further, they need to be away from other environmental toxins and pollutants that are present near nuclear plants, coal fired generators, factories, and highly populated areas. Young Living has six

farms on three continents located in remote, clean environments.

3. Distill. Every plant material is different and, therefore, distillation of each plant can have variances. Some plants need to be distilled immediately upon harvesting while others may need to cure for several days. These differences significantly impact the quality of the constituents that contain the therapeutic benefits. Once ready to distill, Young Living's proprietary, low-temperature, low-pressure steam distillation process ensures that each oil is uncompromised during the extraction process.

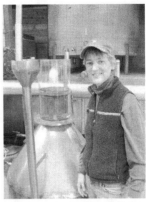

Casey at the distillation of Balsam Fir at St. Marie's Farm in Idaho, 2012.

4. Test. Young Living oils must pass stringent testing to ensure the optimal bioactive compounds are present. Internal and third-party laboratories are used to verify purity and each essential oil is tested during various stages. Young living has been able to compile and categorize over 280,000 references to build their own library for uncontested plant identity.[53]

---

[53] Young Living Essential Oils Product Guide, 2011, p. vii.

5. <u>Seal.</u> Young Living completes the Seed to Sealä process by carefully filling each bottle at its own high-tech, state-of-the-art production facility. Only after each bottle is sealed and inspected is it ready to be shipped.

In an industry that is typically more concerned with profit margins than the quality of essential oils that end up in a bottle, you might be wondering why Young Living goes through such rigorous steps and follows such strict standards. Dr. Young's personal story explains why:

> "Following a painful and debilitating accident, Gary Young began searching for natural alternatives to traditional medical treatments. After being given some research papers on essential oils that were written by French medical doctors and translated into English, he began his quest for further knowledge about the therapeutic properties of essential oils. Through this research, Gary ventured down a whole new path of healing.
>
> Growing up farming, Gary had great interest in learning how to grow and harvest herbs and plants for the extraction of the oils. He developed a proprietary design and technique of distillation for his own essential oil production.
>
> The developing farms, his amazing research discoveries from ancient history to present-day science, and the phenomenal results from his

clinical trials and studies with oil usage encouraged and promoted the beginning of his lifelong mission: to bring this forgotten knowledge back to the modern world."[54]

Today, after over 20 years of dedication to building the company and the brand, Young Living offers over 300 essential oils and essential oil products. Whether it is skin care, personal care, kids products or nutritional supplements, every single product is infused with essential oils to maximize its effectiveness.

In addition, Young Living has accumulated the collective experience and wisdom of thousands of therapists and users over the past 20 years.

Walk the talk

If you are like many consumers you might be skeptical about this Seed to Seal process, wondering if it really exists. The answer is "Yes," and the proof is available for the public to experience. As passionate users of

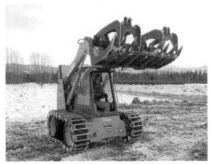

Casey working at the Winter Harvest in Highland Flats, Idaho, 2012

the Young Living product, Alan and I have personally

---

[54] Young Living Essential Oils Product Guide, 2011, p. iv.

participated in the process. Young Living lets its customers and members volunteer throughout the year in the planting, harvesting, and distillation of oils at their farms. In fact, they encourage it specifically so people can see all the incredible work that goes into making pure, therapeutic grade essential oils.

So, next time you go to the store to buy an essential oil, ask yourself these questions:

- Does this manufacturer invite consumers to be part of their planting, harvesting, or distillation process?
- Do they allow you to visit their manufacturing plant where you can physically see the oils being bottled?
- Are they currently using their oils as U.S. FDA & Australian TGA approved internal supplements?

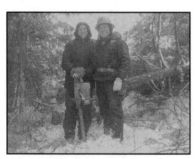

Alan cutting down trees with founder, Gary Young, at the Winter Harvest in 2011.

If the answer to these questions is, "No," then you want to consider why you are using that product. Do you really want to put something on or into your body when you aren't sure of the source? If you are like most people who are still reading at this stage of this publication that answer is easy—No!

Why such an endorsement?

Because we are advocating Young Living products, it is natural for readers to stop and question, "So, why are these authors endorsing this one essential oil company? What's in it for them?" Yes, the authors both use the Young Living products and are independent distributors of the product, but the goal of this book is simply to educate.

There are thousands of Young Living distributors around the world who have no connection with us and whom you can directly contact about purchasing these products. The reason we invested the time, energy and effort into writing the book was because we can only personally educate a small number of people through our lectures, seminars and events. By publishing a book that provides consumers with a basic understanding of how essential oils can fit into your health and wellness goals, we can reach more people and have a greater impact.

By the way, we are not saying that essential oils will be your cure-all for everything or that you shouldn't use modern medicine when necessary. What we are suggesting is that if you have an option to use something that is natural, effective and doesn't

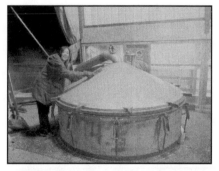

Alan's wife, Linda, keeping the cooker clean!

contain potentially harmful ingredients, WHY WOULDN'T you use those items as a first choice? When integrated with a healthy lifestyle, the outcomes you will obtain with essential oils can be remarkable.

Chapter 9

Using Oils in Everyday Life

If you have made the decision to begin removing toxins, chemicals, and pharmacology from your life and replace these items with essential oils (and essential oil products), the next logical question is, "Where do I use them in my life?" The answer is everywhere. Whether it be a child's cut or scrape, a burn while cooking, cleaning the house, calming the dog during a thunder storm, or giving yourself a boost of energy during your workout, essential oils can be incorporated into your everyday life and that of your family. Let's discuss some of the more common areas of life where adding authentic grade essential oils can make a difference.

Mom's first aid kit

If the only reason you began using essential oils was for the natural health of your kids then it would be a wise decision. Of course, we have to tell you "You should consult your pediatrician before using essential oils." But if you have children then you have lots of situations every day where you are reaching for traditional medicines and products that contain potentially dangerous chemicals in them. With just a handful of essential oils in your cupboard you will eliminate most, if not all over-the-counter (OTC) drugs you might currently be using. Here is just a short list of the most common "first aid" uses you probably experience on a daily basis:

- **Cuts and scrapes**—Don't reach for Neosporin or hydrogen peroxide! Grab some lavender instead.

- **Sunburns**—Instead of aerosol sprays like Solarcaine that are loaded with chemicals, use Lavaderm (a spray made by Young Living), which will instantly stop sunburn pain naturally and help promote healing. This product also works wonders on any burn. Of course, not getting sunburn in the first place is even smarter!

- **Stomachaches**—Stop using chemical antacids when one drop of peppermint should take the common stomachache away. It can be taken sub-lingual, in a glass of water or even rubbed directly on the stomach.

With just a handful of essential oils in your cupboard you will eliminate most, if not all over-the-counter (OTC) drugs you might currently be using.

- **Aches & Pains**—STOP using liver-damaging Ibuprofen! Simply rub Panaway (a blend) directly onto the spot that has pain. Wintergreen works, too.

- **Sore throats**—Why buy processed sugar-latent lozenges when you can use lemon oil? Add a drop to a cup of hot water with some honey and you not only relieve the sore throat but stay hydrated at the same time.

- **Fevers**—Most people don't think twice about reaching for the liquid Tylenol when their child has a fever, but there is an alternative to these potentially liver-damaging drugs. One drop of peppermint oil on the bottom of a child's foot every hour will usually bring their temperature down.

- **Bug bites**—We all know the dangers that are present in most bug sprays. Sure, you can avoid DEET, but what about all those other chemicals! Bugs hate the smell of Purification (a blend). So, you keep the bugs away and don't have that nasty bug spray smell lingering on you and your clothes. An added bonus is that you can put the kids to bed without worrying about washing the spray off of them.

- **Stress & anxiety**—Whether it is normal everyday stress or perhaps a mid-afternoon melt-down, Peace & Calming (a blend) is sure to take the edge off the moment. This can be diffused, but also works wonders on the bottom of the feet prior to naptime.

- **Immune booster**—When was the last time your entire family went through the winter without colds and flu's? Thieves oil (a blend) is a powerful immune booster. This combination of oils was developed after historical research showing how a band of thieves during the great plague of Europe avoided getting sick while robbing graves because they doused themselves in this powerful set of oils and spices.

- **Stretch marks**—Many mom's end up with stretch marks. They may be a natural consequence of pregnancy but no one wants them! Many women report that a blend called Gentle Baby works wonders on reducing or minimizing stretch marks. (Also reported as great on any scar tissue.) Another product called Claraderm spray is also a popular choice with stretch marks.

- **Menstrual cramps/moodiness**—Whether it is a teenage girl on a roller coaster of new hormones or Mom herself, any woman who has had menstrual difficulties knows it's not fun. (Of course, the guys in the house usually don't find it fun either!) For dealing with the physical pain many women report that peppermint, PanAway and Deep Relief all will either stop or greatly reduce menstrual pain. Another blend called Dragon Time has been reported to also help considerably with the emotional swings many teenage girls and some women experience.

- **Menopausal symptoms**—Hot flashes happen to many women as their body goes through major hormonal shifts during menopause, which can last for years with some women. Clary Sage and SclarEssence essential oils help to support a woman's hormones, resulting in fewer of the highs and lows that are at the root of hot flashes. A product called Progessence Plus Serum has helped thousands of women get through hot flashes without synthetic drugs.

  Recently, we were giving a talk on essential oils and hormones and a woman in the audience began to have a hot flash. She had been quite skeptical throughout the talk, asking a lot of good questions. She raised her hand and said, "I'm having a bad hot flash right now; show me how this stuff works!" She placed one drop of Progessence plus under her tongue and the hot flash immediately subsided. We practically had to pry the bottle out of her hands to get it back!

These are just some of the most common everyday First Aid uses for essential oils. As you deepen your education and application of oils, you will find that there is an essential oil for just about every non-life threatening situation your family may encounter.

Pet care

Please note that when using essential oils with your pets there are some differences in application. Specifically, with small pets and cats the oils needed to be diluted considerably. Because this book is not designed to cover this topic, please visit www.AnimalDeskReference.com for more information. This is the website and resource library of Dr. Melissa Shelton, a veterinarian who has integrated the use of essential oils into her practice and now educates pet owners and vets around the world.

- **Pain**—At some point in the life of your pet you will be faced with an injury. Whether it is because of an extra long hike, arthritis, or a scuffle, when your pet needs pain relief, PanAway will provide it.

- **Anxiety**—Many dogs are hyper-sensitive to thunder and lightning. Others just tend to be "high-strung". This can cause many families frustration and lots of damage to the home. Peace & Calming is a wonderful blend that will bring relief to your pet. Some owners begin diffusing it as soon as the forecast calls for bad weather.

- **Overheating**—If you hike with your dog or have a horse, you know how easily these animals can become overheated. A drop of peppermint helps to bring down their internal body temperature and provide fast, cooling relief.

- **Bugs/parasites**—If you have pets you also have fleas, ticks and mosquitoes and other bugs. Just as the blend Purification was used with people, it is wonderful as a repellent for your pets. Best of all you don't have to use those nasty sprays!

- **Behavioral issues**—Sometimes your pets just don't want to cooperate and at times can even be naughty. Valor helps to calm the animal and help support them without aggression. This oil is used with animal trainers around the world.

- **Dental infections**—As your pets age they often get an abscessed tooth. If you begin using Thieves oil around the tooth that is beginning to discolor, you can prevent or delay the need for extraction. This powerful blend can also be used for acute dental infections because of its strong, anti-bacterial properties.

- **Cysts**—More and more pets seem to be developing masses and cysts. Anyone who has a Golden Retriever can relate to this! Lavender has shown to be a remarkable anti-tumor oil.

- **Hot spots**—This is one of the most common skin conditions for animals. A combination of Thieves, lavender, melrose, distilled water, and rubbing alcohol in a spray bottle will dry up hot spots in 24 hours.

Household

- **Disinfectant**—Instead of using toxic chemicals to wash floors and run dishwashers, use a few drops of Thieves oil blend. The company also makes a complete line of Thieves household cleaners.

- **Odors**—Whether it is from pets, the kids sneakers, or mysterious smells coming from the basement, traditional deodorizers simply mask the odors with chemicals. By diffusing Purification blend oil, you will actually destroy the odors. Use a cotton ball to apply Purification onto air conditioning and heating vents and bring it along to freshen up a hotel room while you travel.

- **Cleaner**—Many of us grew up with the scent of lemon from a variety of household products like furniture polish and laundry soap. Add a few drops of lemon oil into a spray bottle and fill it up with water. Keep this in the kitchen to clean and disinfect your countertops. Add a drop of lemon or Citrus Fresh blend to your washing machine and place a few drops of lavender oil onto a facecloth and let it run through the dryer with your clothes. Now you won't need chemical saturated dryer sheets to have fresh smelling laundry!

Athletic performance

- **Energy**—Everyone wants more energy, and we often reach for high-calorie sports beverages or caffeinated energy drinks. All are loaded with chemicals. Natural energy is simple; place a drop of peppermint oil underneath your tongue. This oil is an oxygenator and will give you the boost you need.

- **Athlete's foot**—If you have ever suffered from athlete's foot you know how horrible this fungus can be and how difficult it is to cure. But, preventing (and treating) athlete's foot is actually quite simple: rub lemon oil onto the feet each night. It prevents the fungus from happening plus makes your feet smell good.

- **Overheating**—For endurance athletes or even kids running around the soccer field on a super hot day, overheating is common. Adding peppermint oil to water is helpful in bringing down your internal body temperature quickly.

- **Muscle aches/pain**—Overtraining is a normal part of being an athlete, but it doesn't make it any easier! Deep Relief, which is a roll-on blend of oils, is fantastic for relieving muscle aches and pains. Individually, wintergreen and peppermint oils are wonderful, and when combined they pack a powerful punch.

  - **Lower back**. 75% of adults in western society are expected to visit a medical care professional for back pain at least once in their lifetime. As both authors have faced serious back issues, we know all too well that back pain can be most debilitating. For spasms, use basil essential oil. For pain, you can try any of the oils suggested for general aches/pains above as well as PanAway, Aroma Siez and Relieve It blends.

- ○ **Knees/hips**. One of the fastest growing medical issues today involves knee and hip replacements. Active Baby Boomers and the increase in obesity have been major contributors. In addition to any of the essential oils for general muscle aches/pains, for joint stiffness and pain you can also blend your own recipe:

  - 10 drops black pepper
  - 2 drops rosemary
  - 5 drops marjoram
  - 5 drops lavender

- Antioxidants—Every athlete knows that any type of strenuous exercise causes oxidation in the body. This is why having a diet high in antioxidants is so important. Fruits like blueberries, raspberries, strawberries, and pomegranates are known to be high on the antioxidant scale (ORAC), with scores in the low 2,000's. Clove oil, on the other hand, has a rating of over one million and seventy-eight thousand on the same scale! By taking one to two drops of clove oil per day, you can give your body the valuable antioxidants it needs to repair itself.

Chapter 10

The Everyday Oils

As you read through the list of how different oils can be used for common, everyday application you may have noticed that many of the oils were listed numerous times. That's great news for new users to oils because with just a handful of oils you can have something in the house for just about any everyday situation.

There are 9 oils that are referred to as the Everyday Oils. For those new to the world of essential oils we recommend that you invest in these, and the company sells it in a convenient set called The Everyday Oils Kit. Below is a listing of each essential oil, a description and a quick reference for some of the common uses. For a nice PDF reference booklet for the Everyday Oils, please visit http://keystoyoungliving.com/everyday

---

With just a handful of oils you can have something in the house for just about any everyday situation.

Frankincense

Frankincense is considered a holy anointing oil in the Middle East where it has been used by nearly every ancient culture for thousands of years. Those who attend Catholic church ceremonies will recognize the scent of Frankincense as it is used in a resin burner during most ceremonies. This oil is stimulating and elevating to the mind and is used by many people during meditation, studying, or other activities that require concentration. There is a lot of research happening at present with Frankincense and cancer treatment. Some of the common uses for Frankincense are:

- For fine lines and wrinkles place this oil in your natural facial moisturizer or apply neat (straight, undiluted) to the desired area. If the natural facial moisturizer is not a cream you could eat then use Frankincense neat or add it to organic coconut oil or Young Living V6 oil. (Remember to be careful not to get essential oils in the eye because it will be uncomfortable for ten minutes. Review safety precautions.)
- Rub on chest to soothe respiratory dysfunction.
- Apply to minor cuts, scrapes and bruises to reduce redness and discomfort.
- Apply to face to minimize oil production and breakouts.
- Rub on gum or adhesives to remove from household surfaces or skin.

Lavender

With its fresh, floral scent, Lavender is considered one of the most universal of all essential oils. Therapeutic-grade lavender oil is highly regarded as a skin and beauty tonic and is found in many skin care products. Often used for relaxation, lavender oil offers balancing properties that boost stamina and energy. Some of the many uses and benefits for lavender oil include:

- Reduce or minimize scar tissue by massaging lavender on or around affected areas.
- Diffuse lavender to help minimize seasonal allergies.
- Rub onto the bottoms of your feet, diffuse or even place a few drops onto a cotton ball and place by your pillow at night to help provide a deeper, sounder sleep.
- Use on burns, cuts and scrapes to help reduce pain and accelerate healing.
- Use on scalp to help reduce or eliminate dandruff.
- Use in your washer and dryer to give clothes a wonderful, fresh scent.
- Rub on your neck to relieve stress and tension.

Peppermint

Peppermint oil is also another oil with many diverse uses. It can be used in a wide variety of applications from pain relief to improved concentration. It is highly regarded in supporting digestion; for centuries people have used peppermint tea to soothe a stomachache. Just one drop of pure, therapeutic grade peppermint oil is the equivalent of 28 cups of tea! Some of the more common uses of peppermint include:

- Add to a glass of water for stomachache.
- Add to water throughout your day as a digestive or to aid in the relief of constipation.
- For fever relief, place a drop of peppermint on the back of your neck and on the bottom of each foot.
- If you have a headache simply place a drop of peppermint onto the area of your head where the pain is stemming from.
- For muscle aches apply peppermint directly onto the affected area. For additional relief first apply wintergreen.
- If you have any sinus congestion, place two drops of peppermint into the palms of your hands, rub them together in a circular motion three times and then bring your cupped hands up to your nose. Close your eyes and breathe deeply for 60 seconds.

Lemon

Lemon essential oil has a pleasant, purifying, citrus scent that is revitalizing and uplifting. And, it just doesn't smell good; it's also a powerful germ fighter. Hundreds of hospitals in Europe use it in lieu of bleach. Some of the common uses for lemon are:

- Diffuse Lemon oil to protect your home form airborne bacteria.
- Put a drop in your drinking water for extra vitamin C and to give your body valuable limonene, an antioxidant.
- Use to remove household stains. Place 10-15 drops into a gallon (3.7 liters) of water to remove stains from carpet.
- Disinfecting countertops and use in your laundry.
- Can be used as a toner for oily skin.
- Mist fruits and vegetables with lemon oil water to preserve shelf life.

Thieves®

The Thieves® blend is founded on the legend of a group of thieves in fourteenth century France who used clove, rosemary and other aromatics while robbing plague victims in order to stay immune and healthy. This oil blend is a powerhouse for your body's defense system and will help your family avoid sickness—especially during the cold and flu season. Some common ways in which people are using the Thieves® blend include:

- Diffuse in your home for 15-minutes per day to eliminate bacteria and odors from the air.
- Place on the bottom of your feet to help keep your immune system strong.
- Place a drop of oil in a teaspoon of honey to soothe a sore or scratchy throat.

- Gargle with one drop into an ounce of water for several days after any dental procedure to accelerate healing and minimize infections.
- Add one drop to your dishwasher or laundry to eliminate bacteria and odors.

The Thieves blend oil actually has an entire line of products that include hand soaps, antibacterial gel, household cleaners and dental products. For a free booklet on the entire Thieves line by Young Living, please visit http:// keystoyoungliving.com/thieves

Peace & Calming®

This popular oil blend contains tangerine, ylang ylang, blue tansy, orange, and patchouli. As its name suggests, this blend contains properties that relax the mind, calm the body and promote a deep sense of peace. Some ways in which people enjoy using this blend include:

- Diffusing in the bedroom to promote a deep, restful sleep.
- Placing a few drops into a spray bottle with water and misting pillows and sheets. This is a great option if you don't have a diffuser.
- To calm hyperactive children or pets when traveling use the spray bottle technique in the car.
- Rub a few drops under the nostrils to help reduce snoring.

- Wear on neck, wrists or behind ears prior to boarding a plane. Not only will you feel calmer but your travel companions will reap the benefits as well.

PanAway®

PanAway® is a soothing essential oil blend containing eugenol, a constituent used historically to numb gums when experiencing a toothache. Also containing wintergreen and clove—two oils traditionally used for pain relief—this oil blend aids the body's natural response to irritation and injury.[55] Gary Young created PanAway® after a severe injury to the ligaments in his leg. Some common ways in which people use this oil are:

- Apply to head or neck area to alleviate a headache.
- For broken bones or pulled muscles, apply to the affected area.
- For menstrual cramps apply directly onto lower abdomen.
- When getting a massage, have practitioner add several drops to the V-6 blend or other Young Living massage oil base.
- For back pain, rub several drops into the area of the spine that is affected.
- If going on a long hike, standing on your feet or travelling for long hours, rub PanAway® on your feet.

---

[55] This statement has not been evaluated by the Food and Drug Administration.

Purification®

Purification® blend contains citronella, rosemary, lemongrass, lavandin, melaleuca alternifolia, and myrtle. It was formulated for diffusing to cleanse and sanitize the air and neutralize mildew, cigarette smoke, and other unfavorable odors. However, it can also be used directly on the skin to cleanse and soothe insect bites, cuts and scrapes. Some of the common uses for Purification® include:

- Diffuse in areas of home where mildew smells are common.
- Diffuse in office area where air conditioning ducts are not in your control.
- Use a cotton ball to place oil onto air conditioning and heating vents both at home and when you travel and are staying in hotel rooms.
- Apply to any type of bug bite to reduce swelling and redness. If you get bit by a spider you should immediately seek medical attention.
- Apply to the head of a tick found on your person or pet and watch the tick back out by itself, ensuring the head does not lodge into the skin.
- Add Purification® to a spray bottle with distilled water and spray on your pet prior to going outdoors. This helps repel ticks, fleas and mosquitoes. For increased effectiveness, add several drops of peppermint to this spray.
- Apply to blemishes to help clear skin.

Valor®

This blend contains spruce, blue tansy, rosewood, and frankincense. Valor® is an empowering blend that promotes feelings of strength, courage, and protection. It has also been found to support energy alignment in the body, gaining the respect of chiropractors. Common uses of this blend include:

- Rub onto bottom of feet to help align and balance the body systems.
- Put on wrists to ease anxiety and yield confidence and courage. Mother's have reported using this with their children prior to recitals, concerts and athletic events.
- Massage onto neck, chest and shoulders to relieve tension.
- For those suffering from back pain or conditions like scoliosis, rub onto spine.
- For children who have ADD or ADHD, put a drop of Valor® on each foot before leaving for school.

Below is a link to a movie Young Living produced some years ago, but in 8 minutes it gives a wonderful overview of each of those oils and has some words by Gary Young about essential oils. If you have the time it is well worth watching.

http://bit.ly/PDwAB8

The 9 Everyday Oils are the perfect kit to start with on your journey into essential oils. Whether you need something for your body, your mind, emotions, or around the home, these oils will serve you well every time.
http://keystoyoungliving.com/everyday

Chapter 11

How to Get Started

For most people, the world of essential oils is totally new and, although they like the concept and believe using natural products is a better alternative to chemicals and drugs, they don't know where to start. Perhaps the easiest way to get started is to invest in an Everyday Oils kit, which provides you with the 9 essential oils that were outlined earlier. As the name implies, these kits provide you with something for just about any situation you and your family will encounter in everyday life.

Some people have a specific reason they are learning about essential oils. In that case we have found that most people fall into four categories of need.

1. Immediate physical concern. This is the category of person who is most motivated to start using essential oils because they are having a problem. Whether they aren't getting relief with traditional options or they are seeking natural alternatives to begin with, or, when someone has a pain or has discovered an illness, they usually want to act fast. If you fall into this category then choosing the

essential oils or products that you need is relatively simple. Use the online resources we outline at the end of this book and make a selection.

2. Challenging emotional concern. This is the category of person who is either personally dealing with emotional issues like depression, stress, anxiety, child's behavioral issues, forgetfulness, lack of concentration, etc. Physically getting the body to relax helps to calm emotions, hence why essential oils work so well with emotions. If you (or perhaps a family member) fall into this category you also want to use the resources we suggested and do some research as to which oils would be most beneficial to support that emotional concern.

    Next, we suggest either going on-line to the Young Living catalog and reading through the essential oil blends to see a) which oil resonates best with you, and b) to cross-reference the individual oil ingredients with the list you established with your research. For example, if you are stressed and are having difficulty sleeping, the blend Peace & Calming would be an excellent choice. The company also makes a wonderful roll-on called Stress-Away. Only by reading the descriptions will you be able to make a determination yourself as to which oil is best suited for your particular needs.

3. Removing chemicals & toxins. This category of person may be interested in preventative health

due to recently learning the potential dangers of all the chemicals and toxins in our daily use and environments. Alternatively, this person may be experiencing symptoms like rashes or perhaps even neurological conditions that have been linked to toxicity in the body and may be considering the use of essential oils in the detox process. The latter is obviously more serious. In either case these individuals first need to re-read the earlier sections of this book and then take a serious inventory of the household and personal care products they are using and begin removing and replacing them with natural, chemical-free products.

4. Prevention. This category of person has been introduced to the world of essential oils, doesn't have any major emotional or physical concerns, might even live a 'green' lifestyle now, but wants to incorporate essential oils for healthy living. For these individuals we suggest looking at the Everyday Oils Kit discussed earlier. Evaluate personal care and household cleaning products and begin to remove potentially harmful items. Doing this now could prevent medical issues and conditions in the future.

Non-negotiables!

Although most of our time in the second half of this book has been spent discussing essential oils, we want to re-emphasize the importance of removing harmful toxins and chemicals from your personal care and household products. This is an important part of the wellness process.

Think about this: you can eat well and even use essential oils, but if you are constantly putting toxins back into your body you won't get the best results. When people ask us where to start in this category it is simple. We call them the "non-negotiables", and it means exactly what it says. It is absolutely imperative that you immediately—at a minimum—remove the following harmful items from your home and personal use products (assuming they have one or more of the chemicals we discussed earlier) and replace them with all natural products:

1. Shampoo
2. Soap
3. Toothpaste
4. Deodorant

Check the labels on each of these items. If they have any petrochemicals in them (Sodium lauryl sulfate, propylene glycol and/or DEA) you need to make a change. If you have decided to begin using essential oils, add these personal care items to the list of essential oils you want to purchase. Not only are all Young Living products all-natural, but remember you get the added benefit of essential oils being infused in every product.

Live by this motto: "If you won't eat it then don't put it on or in your body!"

How to get products

Up to now we have intentionally left out any information on how you would go about getting your products should you make the positive decision to start using essential oils. We used to take this same approach in our seminars because we wanted attendees to feel completely comfortable and not feel compelled to buy. However, we found that people preferred that we give them the information so they didn't have to contact us to get it at a later time.

Young Living products are not available in stores, but you can purchase all of the products online. You have two options; you can be a retail member and pay retail prices or you can invest $40 and become a wholesale member, which gives you a 24% discount on all your purchases.

Regardless of which option you take, Young Living is a member referral program. This means that you will need to have the member number of someone when you place your first order. If a Young Living distributor was the one who introduced you to this book you will find their membership number on the inside cover of this book. If you purchased this book online (in either digital or an actual printed book), you can use member #1070785 when prompted.

Ordering Resources

We find that most people who go onto the Young Living website to place an order contact us with a couple of common questions. Below are the links to several videos that answer common ordering questions.

The first short video explains to you the two different membership options you have; straight customer or discounted wholesale. This is worth a quick listen because it clears up any confusion as to the difference between wholesale and retail.

http://bit.ly/AccountTypes

These next two videos actually walk you through a live on-screen recording of how to set up your Young Living Account. If you have chosen to take advantage of wholesale prices (24% discount) then you will want to watch the first link. If, however, you want to pay retail prices watch the second link.

http://bit.ly/WholesalePrices

http://bit.ly/RetailPrices

If you want to just go onto the Young Living website to have a look around, their URL is: www.YoungLiving.com

Remember, no matter which type of account you set up, you will need a member number (called sponsor and referrer). If you have not been given a number by another member you can use ours, which is: 1070785*

*If you purchased or received this book from a Young Living member, please check the inside cover for their membership number.

Chapter 12

Frequently Asked Questions

For those who have used this book as a reference rather than reading it from cover to cover, below is a short list of the most frequently asked questions for an individual new to essential oils. All of these questions have been addressed throughout this book in greater detail. Please see the table of contents to find appropriate sections.

- **Are essential oils safe to use?** When using pure, therapeutic grade essential oils they are safe SO LONG AS you follow the safety guidelines. Please see the earlier section that outlines precautions.

- **Can I use essential oils on kids and infants?** Many people around the world use essential oils on kids and infants. Often dilution is recommended, so please educate yourself on various essential oils, uses and dosing instructions before using on your children.

- **Can I use essential oils on pets?** Veterinarians who practice natural medicine use essential oils on all kinds of pets. Some animals require significant dilution—especially smaller animals. For proper use of essential oils with your pets, please refer to www. animaldeskreference.com.

- **Can I mix different types of essential oils together?** Yes, by mixing certain essential oils together you can create a synergistic blend. This is why many blends already exist. Do your homework on which oils blend better, mix fewer oils to start, and test for effect. Finally, follow your nose and simply identify whether or not you like the smell.

- **Where do I apply an essential oil?** The general rule is that for a physical issue you apply the essential oil to the area of concern—i.e. if your knee aches put the oil/s on your knee. For aromatic and or emotional support you can place the oil wherever you feel it will suit you best (under your nose, on your wrists, etc.)

- **Is there a limit on the number of essential oils I can put on my body at one time?** There is no limit to the number of oils you can use at once, just be warned that using several oils at the same time can create a strong fragrance that might not be pleasing to some family members, friends or co-workers.

- **Can I "over-dose" on essential oils?** It is conceivable that human beings can overdose on anything. Therapeutic grade essential oils are non-toxic but beware: they are habit forming!

- **Are there any negative side effects with using essential oils?** Initially your spouse/partner/friends may say you smell funny or flowery. J Some oils may feel too warm on your skin (this is referred to as an essential oil being 'hot') and, therefore, you may initially need to dilute certain oils before applying.

- **Can I use essential oils if I am taking a prescription medication?** We are not medical professionals and, therefore, must recommend that if you are on a medication you should do your research by using the reference materials we have suggested and/or talk to your doctor. Please see the testimonial section of this book to read about individuals who may have been on medications and began using essential oils.

- **What is the difference between a "single" and "blend" oil?** A single consists of only one type of essential oil (lavender, lemon, peppermint, etc.), whereas a blend is typically three or more essential oils that have been combined for a specific application or effect.

- **What does 'neat' mean in relation to using oils?** This refers to the use of an essential oil topically and without dilution—"straight-up".

- **What does the term "adulteration" mean in relation to an essential oil?** Adulteration is a term used when something has been added to a pure essential oil or it has been altered during a processing step. Filler oils or synthetic fragrances are common additive culprits. The reason it happens is because manufacturers want to make more money. ANY alteration of an essential oil voids it from being considered therapeutic grade.

- **An essential oil bottle at the store says 100% oil, but it does a lot less than the same Young Living oil; why is this?** Essential oils are regulated by the FDA under perfume industry guidelines. As a result the packaging labels can be very misleading to customers. A bottle can say 100% pure oil on it because it is all oil—but often it includes filler oil. The only way you can know you are buying essential oil that is 100% therapeutic grade is by knowing the exact standards and methods that were used in the entire process. Young Living's Seed to Seal™ process gives you total assurance that what you are buying is the absolute best essential oil.

- **Since everybody claims their oils are better, how do I know which oils are truly therapeutic?** Technically, the only way you will really know if an oil is pure, hence therapeutic, is by having it tested in a lab, which isn't going to happen. Therefore, as a consumer there are several things you can do to determine the quality and grade of an oil. First, research the company; are they only a bottler buying oils from the marketplace? Do they grow plants but not have their own distillation process? And, if they say they are in control of every aspect from growing to bottling can they prove it? Second, use the smell test. If a seller has sample bottles compare them. Anyone who compares a bottle of Young Living to a store brand immediately smells the difference. Finally, by using the product. IF you have done all the research, determined the essential oil is therapeutic, and feel comfortable testing it, the only question left is, "does it work"?

- **Why is there a big difference in price between essential oil brands?** Essential oils that are pure, therapeutic grade are more expensive because they are a quality product. You do get what you pay for. If two oils are vastly different in price it is likely that the less expensive one is adulterated. Your nose can tell the difference!

- **I'm overly sensitive to perfumes and fragrances. Will essential oils bother me?** Many people who are sensitive to perfumes and fragrances are actually having a reaction to the synthetic materials in these products. This is why many people will get a "perfume headache" when in department stores. Although some people initially find certain essential oils "strong" they do not usually cause any headaches. In fact, the reverse is true—a headache will usually disappear when pure, therapeutic grade oils are inhaled. Individuals with sensitive

noses should use one oil at a time until they are
accustomed to the aromas.

- **Why do I seem to be attracted to some oils yet
  dislike the smell of others?** For some people certain
  smells bring back particular memories (good or bad).
  In addition, some people initially dislike smells of
  essential oils that elicit certain feelings. For example,
  if you harbor bad feelings you may not like the blend
  Forgiveness. Conversely, if you are consciously
  trying to work on forgiving someone you may be
  attracted to that same blend. The interaction between
  the human mind and body is complex!

- **What is a credible source of information about how
  to use the oils and blends?** In the chapter Educational
  Resources we have explained several credible sources.
  The most comprehensive and easiest to use is the
  Essential Oil Pocket Reference Guide from Life
  Sciences Publishing. http://bit.ly/NzC1EV

- **The Essential Oil Pocket Reference Guide
  gives me multiple suggestions of oils to use for
  a particular situation. How do I choose?** The
  simple answer is "trial and error." You cannot put
  the "wrong" oil on. You may just not put the "right"
  one on for the desired effect. Blends are a great way
  to start because there are several oils in one bottle
  all designed to fulfill the "given name"; Purification,
  PanAway, M-Grain, etc.

- **How can one essential oil have so many different medicinal applications?** Primarily, because single essential oils can have hundreds of naturally occurring compounds. These compounds fall into different categories and have different chemistries that have a variety of medicinal and/or therapeutic effects. Every human body has unique chemistries as well. Therefore, one oil may work wonders for one person and have no effect on another.

- **When I read through the Young Living catalog it only states historical uses for oils and doesn't give the same type of medicinal applications as the Pocket Reference Guide. Why is the company not allowed to put those possible uses in any of their materials?** The simple answer is for legal reasons. Essential oils are mostly recognized for flavoring and aromatic purposes, not medicinal applications. If any product (natural or otherwise) makes a claim about their product—i.e. "This oil reduces pain or inflammation", they will then be regulated by the FDA drug guidelines. Keep in mind that drug manufacturers have the deep pockets necessary to go through this process and it results in a patented product that they will sell through medical doctors and pharmacies and make millions. Essential oils are not patentable because there is nothing proprietary about them; they are the essence of the plant. It would be impracticable for essential oil manufacturers to put themselves through this process so it is just easier to not make any medical claims.

Chapter 13

Educational Resources

One of the most important things you need to learn with essential oils is how to find the answers you need when deciding which oil to use. This is the biggest challenge for most people because, unlike an over-the-counter medication that says "Take two of these capsules every 6 hours", or "apply to burn and cover", there are no instructions with your essential oil bottles. Although this can be challenging for some people in the early stages, once you become familiar with the wonderful resources that are available, your comfort level increases and you quickly begin to grow in your knowledge of what to use in which situation. There are many resources but there are a few key ones that are best for those new to using essential oils.

First, is the *Essential Oil Pocket Reference Guide*. This is a smaller version of a publication called the *Essential Oil Desk Reference*, which would be the equivalent to the *Physicians Desk Reference* (PDR) in the medical world. The smaller guide is perfect to have in your home because you can either look up an oil to learn more about it or you can look up a condition and read through recommendations. For example, you can look up "Poison Ivy" and it will tell you what oils are best. An added benefit is that in addition to the oils, this publication also gives recommendations for nutritional supplements made by Young Living. For most people having this reference is a must. The link to the company that sells it is below and the cost is around $24 plus s/h. http://bit.ly/NzC1EV

Second, we provide our readers and those interested in essential oils with weekly educational tips. These short tips are designed to give you simple, everyday applications that you can refer to and even pass along to friends and family members. We only send tips, no sales stuff, and you can register to receive these here: www. http://keystoyoungliving.com.

Third, it is good to learn how to do a Google search for answers. There are many holistic practitioners who have fabulous blogs on Young Living oils. Some will be very specific, such as entire blogs on the use of oils with your pets while others will offer a variety of topics relating to essential oils. To do a search, go to the Google browser and type in "Young Living + _____". Fill in the blank with what you want to find. For example, "Young Living + seasonal allergies." As you would imagine, following this same process on YouTube will accomplish the same type of search and provide you with video content. Although both of these take some time, you will begin to learn more and more about oils.

Fourth, there is a wonderful website, www.Oil-Testimonials.com. This site is packed with thousands of testimonials from people all over the world who have successfully used essential oils for every situation. So, similar to a Google search, you go onto the site and type in the keyword for the information you want. If you want to discover what others have done for hot flashes you would simply type in "hot flashes." Best of all, it is a free service and only requires you to establish an account by giving your name and e-mail. The only time they will ever e-mail you is if someone posts a new testimonial for a keyword you have searched, which is actually kind of nice.

Fourth, Alan Simpson, co-author of this book, has a large number of free educational resources on his personal website www.AlanYoungLiving.com. These include audios, videos and articles. You can also register there to receive educational tips through his Facebook page.

Of course, if you go to your local bookstore or shop on-line you can find many books about essential oils, but we find that with the Pocket Desk Reference and these free Internet resources you will be able to answer all of your questions in a short amount of time and at a minimal investment, if any.

Summary

Somehow *Vibrant Health Now!* made it into your hands. Whether you read it from cover to cover or simply flipped through to find the pages that most interested you, we hope that you have received enough information to motivate you to make some lifestyle changes and to begin incorporating essential oils and essential oil products into your day-to-day life.

Yes, we are huge advocates today but, just like you we started out knowing nothing about essential oils or how to use them. You can read lots of educational materials, but discovering the wonders of essential oils is an experiential journey that only you can make the decision to take. Therefore, we will leave you with one short phrase, "Let the journey begin"!

We hope you continue with the last section of this book, which is filled with inspirational and interesting stories of everyday people who were introduced to essential oils and ultimately how the oils changed their lives. Maybe someday you can submit a life-changing story of your own.

Testimonials

If you are new to essential oils the best way to realize their incredible benefits is by having your own experience with them. However, hearing how other people have used essential oils is a wonderful way to learn about their application as well as gain a deeper appreciation for their power. On the pages that follow are essential oil testimonials from individuals around the world. They have submitted their story simply to share and received no financial consideration at all.

Below is a grid that lists the person's first name and specific ways/situations where they used essential oils.

Hilary Fournier, East Providence, RI, USA

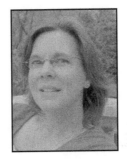

I was introduced to Young Living Essential Oils at a small dinner gathering. My hostess, Casey Conrad, had some friends in town who were distributors and have great knowledge and passion for the oils. They began speaking about the frequency of the oils and our body's frequency. I was fascinated and wanted to learn more. I had been searching for many years for a solution to my low energy levels. I signed on as a distributor and have been experimenting with the oils ever since. For the first time in my life, I am sleeping better and have more energy to keep up with a hectic pace of handling four children and many part time jobs.

I began switching out the oils for products I use on a daily basis. I now clean my face, brush my teeth and use the oils as deodorant. My favorite oil is Abundance. Every time I put it on, opportunities to earn some extra income come my way. I don't know how it works, but it does work.

I saved quite a bit of money on what would have been an expensive visit to our Veterinarian. My cat got a wound that started to abscess. I applied diluted Purification and Lavender oil to the wound a few times a day and massaged it gently in each time. The wound did not seal over and get infected, but continued to drain completely and heal without infection.

My cat was soon back to his old self and I felt very happy to have these wonderful healing oils on hand.

I've used the oils many times for burns, bug bites, acne, aches and pains and allergy relief. Each time I am grateful for a safe and natural alternative. Thank you Young Living Oil for such great products.

Jarrod Stephens, Burleigh Heads, QLD, Australia

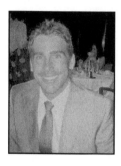
I was introduced to the Young Living oils because of my wife. She wasn't my wife then; I met her and the first thing that struck me was her smell. I thought, "Oh, this is pretty good." I actually said to her, "Wow, you smell unreal. I've never smelled this before." I think she was wearing Stress Away at that time. So, I got introduced to the oils and found my wife at the same time!

Interesting enough, I did not come from a family that did a good job looking after ourselves. We were all very traditional when it came to medical things. If you get sick, take a pill for it. This all changed when I met my wife. Each week she would educate me a little bit more. She never pushed it on me but something would come up from work or sport and I would ask her, "Have you got something for this?" One thing let to another and I opened up a Young Living account for myself because were were only dating at the time.

Although there are many Young Living products I could talk about, the one that has made the biggest difference for me is the enzymes. I had chronic hay fever my entire life. My whole family has it, so I figured between genetics and the region we lived in that it was a given that I would always have the problem. I was always taking antihistamines, four times a day. Other times I would have to take Panadol (ibruprofin) because I was sneezing and itching so much that my face, eyes and tongue would swell up. Sometimes the sneezing would be so out of control that I would get nose bleeds that wouldn't go away. When I was a kid I worked in a fish factory and the combination of the fish, seasonings and cooking would set me off into an attack, then my nose would bleed uncontrollably. It was so bad sometimes that I would have to leave work.

As a Phys Ed teacher hay fever horrible. Not life threatening but debilitating because it can wipe you out for an entire day. It's just like having the flu. Your head gets heavy, your eyes are all red and swollen, your nose constantly drips and you feel like crap. And it can last for a few weeks, depending on how bad the season is.

My wife and I went to the United States for a Young Living convention and heard a lecture on enzyme deficiencies in the body, and they mentioned hay fever as one of the side effects. They also mentioned that diets high in sugar will make hay fever worst. I was willing to try anything so I began taking Essentialzyme and watching my diet. I had been taking the enzymes for about six months when hay fever season hit. I still had some symptoms but it was about 80% better.

About that time the company came out with a new enzyme product called Essentialzyme-4, so I started taking that one as well. Fast forward another year and I went home to visit my family. I'm from Tasmania and the seasonal allergies there are really bad. When I got off the plane and sneezed a couple of times I was a bit worried but that was it. I was there for three weeks and didn't have any problems. No no itchy eyes, no coughing, no itchy throat, nothing at all! What I noticed, however, is that everyone else in my family was getting worse with age. My Dad, who had never had hay fever before, was getting it bad at age 55. And there I was, getting better!

And now my mission is to share this information with others because no one should be suffering from hay fever. Enzymes and avoiding sugar at all cost are critical. I really want to emphasize the elimination of sugars because it compromises your immune system, which adds fuel to the hay fever. I also use certain oils to make sure I don't get any congestion or breathing issues.

The other thing I want to share has to do with hygiene. I am a Phys Ed teacher in the Queensland sun. That means I sweat alot. I used to use regular deodorant several times a day just to keep the odor down. When I found out the bad stuff that was in deodorant I didn't want to use it but couldn't possibly go without something or else people wouldn't be able to stand me by the end of the day. Someone shared with me that if you take a pea sized amount of the Young Living Dentarom Plus Toothpaste and add a couple of drops of geranium oil, which is antibacterial, and smear it under your arms you do not stink. Of course, you still sweat but no smell—even after six hours in the sun running around. In fact, my shirt will be soaked but I could dry it out and wear it the next day if I wanted to. I know it sounds weird using toothpaste but it works great!

Lyn Spinella, Lincoln, RI, USA

My husband, Michael, and I were invited to a very informal kitchen table discussion about health issues at Casey Conrad's home. The get-together was quite casual and that is where I listed to Alan Simpson discuss the great healing powers of essential oils. We left Casey's house that evening feeling enlightened 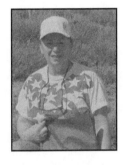 and intrigued enough to look a little more in-depth into the benefits of oils. I signed up that night to be a distributor and looked forward to receiving my starter kit. About a month later, I was hosting a function at my place of business. I was serving BBQ chicken and, as I was removing the dinner from the oven, the disposable aluminum pan collapsed and hot BBQ sauce was spilled all over my lower right leg. Fortunately, I was right next to the sink. It's amazing how high one can lift one's leg when there is a need!! I immediately doused my leg under cold running water but it immediately blistered and the pain was excruciating. I couldn't leave the function so I continued serving my guests and saw the doctor the next day. The doctor looked at my injury and declared it to be burns in the second degree. She prescribed Silverdine and told me to wrap my leg. She also advised that I had to extremely careful that the blister didn't break because of the risk of infection. She also informed me that, unfortunately, this burn would leave a nasty scar. Because I had just learned about the healing powers of essential oils, I decided to go the holistic route. I did some research on line and discovered that Lavender Oil was a good choice for burns. Lucky for me, lavender oil was included in my starter kit! I began by using two drops of Lavender Oil directly on the blister two times daily. With the first application, the pain immediately subsided! I was amazed. Within approximately one week, the flud in the blister had been reabsorbed and the burned skin became a natural band-aid. It was like a vacuum seal had taken place because the once loose skin was now snugly covering the burn. In a total of three weeks, the burn was completely healed and, best of all, NO SCARRING! I went back to the doctor when the injury was healed and she commented that she had never seen a second degree burn heal in such a way! I told her about the Lavender Oil protocol that I used and she completely discounted it and told me that I must be a wonderful healer. Ob well, you just can't convince some people. Since that occurrence, I have become quite active introducing people to essential oils. Both myself and my husband have experienced wonderfully amazing results using essential oils to treat a whole host of maladies.

My husband loves to golf and never thought about using sun protection. In July of last year, he had a biopsy and was diagnosed with skin cancer on his right ear. Thethat doctor set up an appointment six weeks later for a Mohs procedure whereby one layer of skin is removed at a time and put under a microscope. The procedure is repeated until there is no sign of the cancer. My husband came home and started applying one drop of Frankincense to the affected area twice a day. It began to look better, but he kept his appointment for the Mohs procedure. The surgeon took the first layer of skin and brought it to the lab. When she came back, she reported that there was no sign of cancer in the tissue and that the diagnosis must have been incorrect. He told the doctor about the use of Frankincense but again, it fell on deaf ears.

Jadwiga Frankowska, Maryland, NSW, Australia

I had suffered for many years with a skin rash and had been to a number of dermatologists who prescribed lots of different medication, all to no effect so the problem persisted. This has affected me greatly—not just because of the skin, it also disturbed my sleep and had a domino effect. The last skin specialist 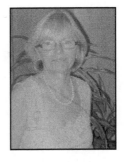 prescribed another medication and told me I needed to be very careful and precise with the dosage, so I asked what he was giving me. He said "Steroids." My reply was

"No thank you! I would rather scratch my body than take steroids.

It was around this time that I met Alan and Linda Simpson and I set up an appointment to have an Indigo Biofeedback reading. During my session Linda told me that in all her years of doing readings she had never seen anyone with such a high percentage of radiation showing up in their body.

When I began to think about my life it became apparent; Chernobyl! I am from Poland and lived there in 1986 when the nuclear plant had the melt down. So, what was happening was the radiation was literally trying to get out of my body through my skin.

This is when I began using Young Living Essential Oils. What I had to do was detox my body, specifically starting with my liver. I began a protocol of NingXia Red, Omega Blue, Longevity capsules, Juva Cleanse Oil and JuvaPower. I also began using several oils, including Helichrysum and Ledum.

As is often the case when I began using the oils my rash actually got worse. A few months into following this specific protocol I got really bad. In fact, my partner called up Alan and said, "I'm a little bit concerned about Jadwiga because, her body has swollen up and is starting leak fluids." This was about 7:30 at night and we live two and a half hour drive away. But Alan said, "I will be right there."

When he arrived he made up an oil blend and wrapped me up in plastic like a mummy. I stayed in that for over four hours. I never had another flair up like that but continued with my protocol. It took 18 months to clear my skin and now you would never know I had such bad skin problems! All the radiation is gone and my skin is beautiful.

I now use all Young Living's products. I love the ART skincare system, the sandalwood cream and I use Joy oil as my perfume, people tell me all the time how young I look, I just smile and say Yes that's because I am using Young Living products!!!

That's my story. I am so thankful for Gary and Mary Young and their wonderful Young Living products.

Louise VonSperl, Castlegrag, NSW, Australia

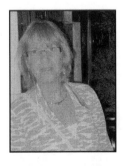

I was introduced to Young Living Essential oils back in 2000 by a friend who does Qigong with me. She asked me to come to a massage workshop featuring the Raindrop technique. Because I used essential oils she said to me, "You'll never experience oils like these" and had me smell how pure and potent they were. So, I bought the Raindrop Kit and signed up to do the weekend event. It was a wonderful event; I enjoyed it and became a believer in the Young Living brand of oils. From then on I began buying only Young Living and using it personally as well as with friends and family.

But it wasn't until a year ago that I had one of those major "Wow" experiences. I had broken my leg; the fibula and a piece of the tibia. The doctor didn't cast it, but put me in a full, orthopedic-leg brace.

He wanted to put me on anti-inflammatories. But I said, "No. I'm going to be using my products that I have with Young Living." The primary thing I was using was Sulfurzyme. At one point I was taking 12-14 capsules per day. I was also taking BLM (bones, ligaments, and muscles) and I increased my Omega Blue consumption. Topically I was putting copaiba, Deep Relief and lemongrass, Dorado Azul, and peppermint. I used a lot of oil multiple times per day.

I also used oils for my emotions. It has been such a nasty fall that I felt off balance for an entire week; almost like I was in shock from the fall. So I used Valor and Peace & Calming to settle me down and also Joy because I felt a little down; I lost my ability to anything myself and was relying on everyone else.

I did this for two weeks and then had my first follow up appointment. The doctor took a new X-ray and he could not believe it was the same person. The bones had repaired so fast that he took the brace off right then. In the hospital he told me I would need to wear it for six weeks and would need 12 weeks to fully recover! I didn't even need to go through any physical therapy, just do my own weight bearing exercises. The entire healing process was accelerated. I was driving within two and a half weeks of the accident. Now that orthopedic surgeon refers his patients to me for the Sulfurzyme.

Of course, the Sulfurzyme has essential oils in it and oils have the same molecular structure as our blood. So every supplement that Young Living makes is harnessing that power. Sure, you can go into any health food store and pick up a fish oil; but it won't have essential oils in it. Further, you don't know who is behind the product. I have actually me the man behind Young Living—Gary Young. This means I know what I am using in and on my body and the integrity of the product. You can't say that with big companies and that is worth a lot to me.

Chris Taylor, Cushing, MN, USA

Like many guys, my introduction to Young Living Essential Oils was through my wife. Although I am thin, I discovered that my cholesterol was 258 and climbing. My stress levels were high and my eating habits not good. My doctor put me on a statin drug and baby aspirin. After six months my cholesterol 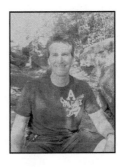 had only slightly lowered. My wife and I decided to try the oils because they are all natural. I informed my doctor and stopped taking the statin drug. However, because I have a family history of cardiovascular disease he didn't want me to stop the baby aspirin. I told him that I wanted to use wintergreen oil instead because it has methyl salicylate, which is the exact same ingredient that's in baby aspirin. His requested documentation on constituents of the pure wintergreen. After analyzing it he okayed the wintergreen in place of the baby aspirin.

Instead I began to do several things with the Young Living products. First, I was drinking four ounces of NingXia Red daily. Second, I began taking the Omega Blue fish oil capsules that have essential oils infused within. Third, I used wintergreen and lemongrass oils. What is interesting about the oils is that I was able to use those for two benefits because I was having ligament and tendon issues with my shoulder. So, I was putting the lemongrass and wintergreen on topically but they were also helping my cholesterol. That's the great thing about the oils—it's not like over the counter drugs that typically only work on one thing.

After six months my cholesterol had dropped from 238 to 201. I continued that exact regimen for a year and it was then time for my annual physical. At that point it had dropped below 200 with my HDL at 62, which is good. It's now going on two years and the only change I have made is dropping the Ningxia Red down to two ounces per day. I can't wait to get my next annual test! I will be going in for my test next, the end of this month, to see where it's at again, another year later.

Young Living Essential Oils are now a part of our daily life. I'm 50 now, have been an athlete my entire life, and I feel as though I'm in my 20's. My energy level is better than ever and I am able to do anything I want. And the health benefits are fantastic.

The entire family uses the oils on a daily basis. One very, very significant change is my daughter's eyesight because of drinking the NingXia red. Prior to using the Young Living products her eyesight had begun to deteriorate. She had gone from perfect vision to 20/60. The doctors thought perhaps it was happening as she was going through hormonal changes. They wanted to send her to a specialist but they never figured out what the cause was. She began consistently drinking one ounce of NingXia every morning before school and taking the True Source Whole Food Vitamins and one year later her vision was 20/10—just two weeks ago. So, all I can say is that Young Living products have really impacted our life.

Cai Wei Boey, Perak, Malaysia

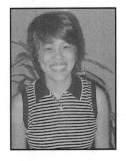

My aunt introduced me to essential oils. When she brought them home I thought they were weird and stinky. Perfumes have always made me dizzy so I avoid them; I figured essential oils would be the same. However, I'm an athlete and frequently twist an ankle or have some other small injury.

With the state championship three months away I seriously injured my ankle. An x-ray confirmed that it was dislocated with torn tendons and cartilage. The doctor said surgery wasn't necessary but I would not be able to walk on it for six months, train for twelve months and that I should not expect to be back into competition form for eighteen months. This was devastating news for me because I had been the State Champion for three years in a row and wanted to go back and defend my title.

My mom was in a panic. She called my aunt, who ordered some oils and explained to us how to apply them. Apply Lemongrass first, wintergreen 2 minutes later, and then peppermint to accelerate the absorption. After applying the oils I would alternate with ice packs and heat for improved circulation and reduction of swelling. In addition I began taking two Young Living supplements BLM and Sulfurzyme. After three weeks of oils and supplements I felt good enough to train and did. Since then I have gone back to competing at the States and have finished in the top ten nationally.

My doctor was in shock. She told us she had never seen anything like that before. In fact, all the physicians said that it wasn't possible. But they worked for me. Now I tell everyone about essential oils. Not only did they help my ankle injury but they have increased my memory a lot and that helps me in school to get better grades.

Atholie Forester, Lake MacQuarie, NSW, Australia

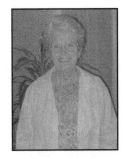

I had a really bad case of shingles on the side of my face and down my eye. Shingles is extremely painful and debilitating, and can affect you for the rest of your life—impairing or even losing eyesight. My doctor had given me drops for it but I wasn't happy with the treatment. I wanted something better.

That is when my friend showed me a book on essential oils; it read like they were magical. I began using an oil called Immupower and two weeks later things began to turn around. Within three weeks the shingles had cleared up. The oil had heightened my immune system, which at that time I discovered was very low. By using Young Living oils I walked away without any side effects! When I went back to the eye specialist he was amazed that my vision was 97% better than it had been a month before.

Today I can say that in every way the oils have given me greater energy. They give you better focus on what you want in your life. In turn you are able to help other people. That is the wonderful thing about sharing the oils. It leads us to such a quality of life, particularly at my age. I'm not a teenager anymore, but I believe I can do a lot more things than other people at my age can do. I'm grateful to have the oils in my life, and grateful for the dedication of the founder, Gary Young.

Susan Johnson, Wakefield, RI, USA

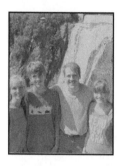

I was introduced to Young Living Oils by my sister. Our family was traveling to New Zealand during the H1N1 flu threat. My husband and I were nervous about traveling in airplanes for close to 35 hours breathing recycled air. We had travelled to Australia several years before and our kids had both gotten sick. There is nothing worse than being thousands of miles away from home and having sick children! She suggested that we put a drop of Thieves on the bottom of our feet for three weeks before we left and while we were away to help our immune system. It worked! None of were sick and enjoyed a great vacation.

My husband and I continued using Thieves after we returned. It was winter and everyone at work and school seemed to be sick. Our kids decided that they did not need to continue. Within two weeks they both got sick. Anyone with kids knows how quickly the entire family can get sick once it is in the house but my husband and I never caught so much as a sniffle.

Fast forward a few years…the whole family, kids included use Young Living products daily. We all have our own favorites. My son uses Clarity and Brain Power, my daughter, Peace and Calming and the ART Skin Care System, my husband lemongrass, Mister, and a variety of enzymes, me, the ART Skincare System, Progessence Plus, Sacred Frankincense and Abundance to name just a few. And of course, we all use Thieves on a regular basis…the oil, the hand soap, the toothpaste, the household cleaner…. We are living a better life thanks to Young Living!

Aaron Bremmner, Naremburn, NSW, Australia

I started using Young Living products for general health. Omega Blues for joint issues, Ninxia Red for cellular vitality and essential oils for my skin. I began to notice small bumps appearing on my fingers. Blister would appear and then my skin would flake off. I thought perhaps it could be a fungal infection 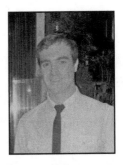 because I had previously worked with fiberglass, polymer glues, and tiling cement. It is not uncommon for people who work with these materials to get fungal infections in their fingernails. What was strange was it had been several years since I had handled any fiberglass.

I began putting Thieves oil on my hands but it didn't seem to help, which was surprising because Thieves blend oil is known to kills bacteria. I then tried lavender oil and noticed that the problem actually spread instead of getting better. It travelled down my fingers and onto my knuckles, palms, and backs of my hands, turning them red and raw. Next I tried I wintergreen, also an antifungal, but it caused my wrists to get inflamed and red.

Finally I went to the doctor. He told me that I had a chemical burn and gave me a silver colloidal cream to use. Soon after the top layer of my skin turned transparent and I could literally see the raw layers underneath. This indicated to me that it wasn't an infection so I decided to go back to the oils.

I started using copaiba and wintergreen but I stopped using the oils because the itch had become too much. Even after stopping the oils the rash and puffiness spread to my elbows, upper arms, and eventually my neck and chest. After a month the lymph nodes on my elbows started oozing a clear, yellow liquid that smelled like the resin I used to work with. I actually had to use compression bandages to stop me from scratching. I continued taking NingXia Red, Omega Blue, and Digest & Cleanse supplements and after a while my skin settled down.

Six months after my skin had cleared up I met a naturopath at a Young Living convention. He explained to me that my skin had absorbed the chemicals and my body had stored those toxins in my fat cells as a protective measure. He recommend that I work my way up to 20-30 Sulfurzyme capsules per day and to use lemon topically to break down the petrochemicals. For three months I took 30 capsules per day and covered myself in lemon oil every time I got out of the shower. I was probably using a bottle of lemon oil per week. I had a few breakouts with some rashes and itchiness, usually when I forgot to take all the Sulfurzyme capsules. After three months I went back down to 10 a day.

In addition to detoxing and clearing up my skin, I noticed several health benefits. First, my asthma virtually disappeared. Now I can go running and rarely have any asthma attacks. If I do I use lemon oil and it settles it down. Second, I don't have dust allergies anymore. Third is that I no longer have a negative reaction to wintergreen oil. When I was detoxing, if I put it on my hand it would puff up and turn red.

Aleena Stephens, Burleigh Heads, QLD, Australia

I was introduced to the oils by my parents, mainly my Dad. He would douse himself daily in oils and I initially thought it stunk! It wasn't the best introduction but that is how it happened.

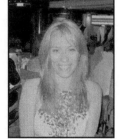

Where my opinion of the oils changes was when I began using oils for my menstrual issues. Specifically I would have severe and debilitating cramps to the point where my Mom would have to come take me out of school. Being an advocate for natural health and healing my Dad was not happy with my taking over the counter pain killers. I had no idea that oils could be used from such things but one day he gave me a capsule of clary sage and peppermint oil as I was walking out the door complaining of the pain.

Although the oils were in a capsule I still had an aftertaste, which was quite unpleasant for me. What I have since learned is that you often don't like the smell or taste of oils that you are most in need of. Obviously I had some kind of hormonal imbalance going on because the clary sage (which is great for women's hormones in general) gave me relief. This really seemed to keep my hormones balanced and mostly prevent the pain.

One of my biggest fears what being somewhere and not having my oils, which is exactly what happened to me while I was attending a Young Living event in Utah. Fortunately I was surrounded by people who had oils and I was able to talk to the founder Gary Young about my issue. Although there were no capsules to be found, Gary had his wife, Mary, put clary sage in some water for me to drink. The taste wasn't very pleasant and made me feel like gagging but I knew it would help.

I continue to use clary sage every month, starting a couple of days before my menstrual cycle. The difference is that now I actually put 15 drops under my tongue and hold it there for five or ten minutes. This sublingual approach seems to work even better. When I follow this protocol I find that I only need to do it once or twice and rarely will

I have any issues. I've also noticed that there's been a significant reduction in the blood flow as well. I also don't seem to get acne breakouts anymore during that time of the month, which is wonderful. The biggest difference, however, is the lack of pain.

Louden & Jenny Grady, Parkes, NSW, Australia

Our introduction to Young Living essential oils came several years before actually using them. A Bowen practitioner colleague of ours called one day and said, "Go to this meeting; you will find it interesting." She didn't say what it was about but out of respect for her we decided to go. Turned out that Jenny couldn't get away but Louden went. The product sounded impressive but for no particular reason I left without buying any oils. Some years later another Bowen practitioner actually used some oils on Louden and he signed up for a kit of oils on the 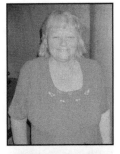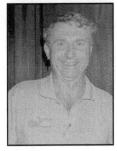 spot. With Bowen therapy you need someone to work on you, where with oils you can treat yourself. Jen wasn't very happy with me so I told her that these six bottles would be enough and we wouldn't buy anymore. Little did I know that she would become the one nagging at me to order more oils! But I'm getting ahead of myself.

We own a horse farm so using the oils on animals was another one of our interests. One of Jenny's favorite horses had previously died of colic. Thousands of dollars of vet bills but nothing could save her. There is nothing worse than losing one of your beloved pets. Soon after getting my oils we had another horse come down with a mild case of colic. I did some research and found that 15 drops of an oil under the horse's tongue was the protocol. In no time the horse was fine.

The real test came about a week later when Jenny's second favorite horse came down with a bad case of colic. We had been off the farm for a number of hours and by the time we found her she was in bad shape. We immediately got a head collar on her and I started to pour the 15 drops of oil into her mouth but after 11 she began to shake her head violently and the last 4 missed. We got her settled down and five minutes later I put the remaining drops in. We stayed with her to observe and about a half an hour later Jen said, "This horse is looking good; it is working well." At three quarters of an hour she took a drink of water and then went and ate some hay! At the hour mark we gave her another dose and then went to bed. It was several months before we could ride her again but she is alive and well. Her case was as bad, if not worse than the horse that died.

Another interesting case is with this one wild cat that our son had tamed. He's like a cat whisperer! Anyway, Muggy, as he was named, gets the cat flu. Our son goes to Louden and says "Muggy is listless and pretty unresponsive and Mom and I are going to take him to the vet." Admittedly the cat looked as if he was within a day of dying, but when you have a bloody barn full of cats Louden said, "No you are not! The only thing we'll have tomorrow is a $500 dead cat." They both expressed what they thought of Louden. The next thing that happens is, the cat gets dropped in Loudens lap and told, "You've got the oils. Fix the cat, Dad."

After reading through the oils it was decided that Thieves and peppermint were the choices; one drop on a front paw and the other on a back one. The cat just lied there and eventually we all went to bed. The next morning our son comes in and says, "Dad, Muggy's good, you should see him." High five's all around. But lunchtime comes around Muggy gets presented to Louden again, listless and limp. Not quite as bad as the day before but not looking so good. So we decide to give Muggy another dose. Well, Muggy must have remembered Louden because he just about shredded his shirt and tore bloody strips out of his arms. Now he was the one that needed the oils! We had to hold Muggy down to give him the oils so he obviously wasn't that bad. When we let him out of the towel he did a few circles and then went straight up the sitting room curtains. It took three months before Muggy would even say hello to Louden but he didn't need another oil treatment. Now he won't leave him alone. We think Muggy knows he saved his life.

One personal story had to do with spider bites. Louden was out working with long pants and work boots on and he got this sharp pain in his foot; felt like a thistle or a seed got into his sock and was sticking into the bottom of his foot. That night he went to bed and didn't think anything of it. When he went to put his boots on the next morning he noticed three little spots on my foot that were puckered up. He quickly thought, "I wonder what that was," but put his socks and boots on and went back to work. When he took my socks off that night the flesh was totally rotting and falling off just by touching it.

He said to Jen, "I think -- that must have been a white tail spider that bit me." He immediately put two or three drops of purification on the area and did that for several days. He ended up having to use some other melaleuca (tea tree) and lemongrass oils to detox the poison out of his lymph glands but didn't have to go to the hospital or use any traditional medical treatments. What is most interesting is that we later ran into a woman who had been bitten by a white tail spider on her wrist and she had treatments and skin grafts over a four year period! That is how serious the bites can be so that makes the oils even more impressive.

Cynthia Shelton-Barrett, Charleston, WV, USA

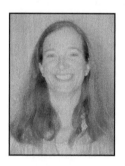

I was introduced to essential oils by my chiropractor, who I actually use as almost a general practitioner. I am a registered nurse but haven't practiced in 14 years since my husband and I started our family. One day I was at the chiropractor and my son was with me. At the time he was five. He had a funny little spot on his shoulder but I couldn't make out what it was. He hadn't scraped it or fallen so I asked the doctor to take a look at it.

Testimonials

I was shocked when she said, "Oh. That's MRSA."
Methicillin-resistant Staphylococcus aureus. I didn't
believe it but she took out her iPhone and pulled up pictures
showing all the different presentations of MRSA. There
it was! The mark on his shoulder was almost identical; it
looked like an abrasion that had gotten puffy and red.

I was not happy because both of my older daughters had
been going through bouts of MRSA for the previous three
months and theirs had just cleared! Apparently they picked it
up from swim lessons at a university pool. The treatment they
went through was horrible. Huge amounts of antibiotics both
internally and topically. Antibiotics are like a nickel bomb
in your stomach; they kill the good with the bad. In addition
they had to lance the MRSA first and I had to change their
bandages three times a day. The school was so terrified that
they made them walk around with Lysol, to spray!

So, our daughters had gone through all—and we had
seemingly just gotten over it—I said, "Oh, my Lord. I can't
do that again." And the doctor said, "You know, it's real
funny. I just got these oils. And I'm kind of using my patients
as guinea pigs. Would you be okay with me trying one on
him? There's this one oil called Thieves. It is killer on staph.
And I've never had anybody with MRSA before. But do you
mind if I try it on him?" I said, "Go for it." And then I looked
at my son to make sure he was okay with it. Of course, he
saw what his sisters had gone through and said, "I'll take an
oil over that any day." So she put Thieves oil on. It stung so
she immediately put some lavender on. It was still stinging
so she tried Gentle Baby and the sting went away completely.

I went home with a bottle of Thieves oil in hand and put one drop on the area three times a day. After about five or six applications it went away completely and never came back. It also didn't sting nearly as much each subsequent time, which made Ned happy. As you can imagine, I went back into the chiropractors office and said, "I need to know more about these oils." I went onto the website and immediately ordered the Thieves Kit.

What was very interesting was that one of my other daughters got MRSA one more time. She had seen what had happened with my son and was thrilled to know that she could use the Thieves, which she did and it cleared up quickly.

Now I actually am building a business with Young Living products!

Naomi Dyer, Camden South, NSW, Australia

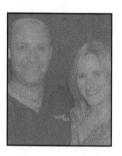

My family was introduced to the oils when our then 8 year old daughter had been suffering from food intolerances from the age of 3. We had put her through many different medical tests, including blood tests and hospital stays. After all of this and with nothing that would help her, it was a parent's nightmare. It was also horrible for her because it was affecting her daily life. She would have an episode at school and end up doubled over in pain and often we would have to collect her from school. She had trouble attending friends birthday parties as should couldn't eat any of the food they were serving, and if she did we would have to leave early. After five years of this cycle, the only solution her pediatrician came up with was giving us a prescription for a strong migraine medication, and telling me "I think it's a rare stomach migraine. When she gets the next one, just give her one of these, and we'll see how it goes".

My husband and I could not do that to her. This led us to searching natural healing solutions and as well as modifying her diet by eliminating any preservatives and additives. We were also introduced to an amazing naturopath who successfully diagnosed the main cause of her issue. It was this person who introduced us to Essential Oils as a medicinal alternative. The issues have now all been sorted out and on the rare occasion that she does get a stomach ache we put DiGize on, and within 2 or 3 minutes it's gone. Of course we are ecstatic, and yet it pains us to think that had we known about essential oils and natural therapies initially, we could have avoided subjecting her to all those invasive and scary medical tests.

Ever since that introduction Essential Oils have become an integral part of our life. We basically don't have any traditional medications in the house anymore, apart from one I have to take to replace my thyroid that has been removed. If the children get a fever we use peppermint to reduce it, if they get an insect bite we use Purification. If they suffer from a virus or flu we use Thieves. We have also replaced all of our household chemicals with the Thieves product line that is non-toxic for children and pets.

Around the time that we were introduced to the oils I was diagnosed with thyroid cancer. After having surgery to remove my thyroid, I ended up with a rare complication of paralysed vocal cords. I was rushed to intensive care, couldn't speak, couldn't swallow, having issues breathing, and in bad condition. After just over a week one of the vocal cords recovered enough for me to be sent out of intensive care, and then eventually home, and then after about 4 months the other recovered. I did, however, have a very bad incision that was not healing properly. It was raised and red, and the doctor said he may have to do further surgery, but wanted to wait so I could regain some strength.

I decided to give the oils a try. I began putting lavender on the scar three times a day. When I went back to the doctor three months later he was shocked and asked what I had done! I told him I'd used Therapeutic Grade Lavender Essential Oil. He was so impressed he wanted information for his other patients!

Another interesting piece to my story is that I later began rubbing Valor and Frankincense on my neck to try and help restore my vocal cords further. Although they were working again, there had been damage meaning that I could not longer shout or sing. Having previously been a professional singer it was difficult to deal with. Since using these two oils I have noticed that I am getting some pitch back, and slowly regaining some of my singing voice, which is fantastic!

Warren Dyer, Camden South, NSW, Australia

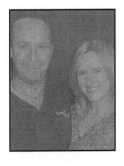

I was introduced to essential oils through my naturopath when our daughter was dealing with food allergies (See Naomi Dyer). My personal story is one of skin cancer. Prior to being introduced to the oils I suffered a lot of skin cancers on my face, which I had to have frozen off regularly. I had one particularly nasty one growing on the side of my nose that would not go away with freezing or radiation creams. After some further testing, the doctor determined that it was a grade of basal cell carcinoma that needed to be surgically removed, so I had it cut out. They also had to do a skin graft on my nose after taking out the cancer. Several months later, I was told I had another one growing right under my eye, and because it was the same type of cancer, it would require the same sort of surgery.

Due to the location of this surgery I was required to sign all sorts of indemnity forms saying that I understood that if they accidentally damaged my eye, it wasn't their fault! It was about this time that we were introduced to the oils, and my naturopath advised me to try Frankincense and Balsam Fir Essential Oils, a few times a day, for a couple of weeks. So, that is what I did. I used one drop each of Balsam Fir and Frankincense oils, 3-4 times a day. I left them in the bathroom so every time I went in there I would remember to re-apply. I also had two other, smaller skin cancers, so now three in total that I was applying the oils to.

Three weeks later, I went back to the skin doctor and ALL of the cancers had gone. Even the major one under my eye. Of course, my doctor just looked at me with that very skeptical look and said "We'll just keep an eye on it, won't we?" That was well over 18 months ago now, and they haven't resurfaced again. Although I couldn't change it, I kept thinking to myself, "If I had been introduced to Young Living Essential Oils just six months beforehand, I could have saved myself major surgery and a lot of discomfort.

Today our family doesn't have a medicine cabinet; we have a 'wellness chest' and it is full of Young Living Essential Oils and products. I carry my oils with me everywhere; in my car, at work, and on holiday. I hand out oils to friends and work associates to help them. Basically, Young Living Essential Oils changed our lives and now we love to share them with others.

Carrie O'Donahue, Molong, NSW, Australia

I was introduced to Young Living Essential oils through my massage practice. There is a technique called Raindrop that I had learned so I could offer it to my clients. I hadn't been using the oils personally until I ruptured

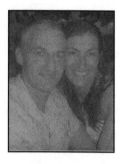

my Achilles tendon. I had just gotten out of the hospital and the gentleman who introduced me to the oils rang me out of the blue to see how I was doing with them. When he heard about my injury he came right over and brought both his oils and a biofeedback device called the Zyto Compass, which reads your body and tells you which biomarkers are out of balance. It then matches up the imbalance with Young Living products.

The device was amazingly accurate! It identified exactly what I needed at that moment; and not just the physical aspects but my emotional state at the time. My response was, "Get me those oils—NOW!"

Over the next year I was using the oils and other Young Living products regularly. One day I was speaking to a friend of mine who does blood analysis. I asked her, "What is the trickiest case study you have ever done?" She said Candida (when yeast organisms take over healthy bacteria in the body) and Parasites (living beings that live off of another host). I suggested to her that we do a study on these two conditions using Young Living Essential Oils and she agreed.

We created three protocols; group A would do nothing, group B would have Raindrop treatments and group C would take oils internally. Because this wasn't some kind of clinical trial I actually started taking DiGize oil the same day we decided to do this. I was consuming 15 drops in a vegetable capsule three times daily. I had taken two doses before I had my first blood draw.

197

When we looked at my live blood under the microscope it was very interesting. It was very active with normal white bloods cells but you could literally see parasites being engulfed. You could also see how much Candida was in my blood—it was everywhere. My dried blood showed that I had a lot of heavy metal toxicity on the outside of my cells. Interestingly enough, that is how I felt, "heavy."

Being a "get it done" person I looked up in the Desk Reference what oils would work on heavy metals and made up a blend of Tea Tree, Lemongrass, Thyme and Agave sweetener. I ended up taking about 80 drops of oil per day, neat (undiluted) for two or three days.

Well, that obviously was a bit too aggressive because at the end of the first day my middle finder began to swell and I began to get encephalitis up my arm! We got that under control but my hand ending up opening up and lymph was oozing out of my fingers.

What we came to realize was that all my years of being a massage therapist and using baby oil and other adulterated oil products (all petrochemicals) had made me toxic, especially in my hands. The detox continued for about six weeks, which was pretty difficult since I'm a massage therapist. But now my hands are clear and I feel great. In fact, prior to doing this detox my finders were swollen and arthritic. Now my fingers are pain free and are actually thinner.

Perhaps most interesting was our "study." On the 5th day—while my hands were swollen and draining toxins—my blood work was fantastic. So, even though I felt like crap my body chemistry was amazing in terms of the Candida and Parasites.

John O'Donahue, Molong, NSW, Australia

I was first introduced to Young Living Essential Oils after my wife had an injury and began using them. I had seen the amazing results she got that I could see they were definitely an alternative to drugs from the chemist. I had my own opportunity to use them when I got a really bad bout of food poisoning. It

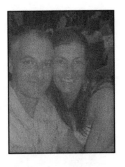

was horrible; I was vomiting, had diarrhea, cramps and a fever. I literally couldn't get out of the bathroom. My wife gave me peppermint oil to put on my stomach and lavender oil for the top of my head. It was incredible; my fever was down within five minutes and within ten minutes all the cramps were gone too. All my symptoms subsided and I was able to go to bed. I woke up the next morning and was fine. I have had food poisoning before and typically you are down for two to three days. But I got up the next morning and went to work like nothing had happened. I, like most guys, can be a bit resistant to these types of things but it was then that I said to myself, "Hmm. There's something about these oils." Personally having that experience made me a believer.

Now I use oils and Young Living products all the time. I have more energy and am open to experimenting with them to just see what works in certain situations. You are constantly learning things about these products.

Suzanne VanOver, West Milford, New Jersey, USA

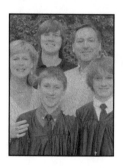

I am a massage therapist and have a client who suffers from Multiple Sclerosis (MS). She came to me with the concern that none of the prescription and over the counter medications were helping her. She was looking for an alternative, hence her holistic approach to specifically address the pain she was experiencing from neuropathy. One day a friend of mind told me that essential oils were good for people suffering from MS. In particular, a technique called "Raindrop" applies a sequence of oils to the feet and spine that can really benefit people neurologically. So I bought a kit of oils and took a class on the Raindrop technique. That was the beginning of my lovely journey into essential oils.

The first time I used the oils with my MS client, it was incredible. I applied the oils to her feet, and she started to cry because it was the first time she had felt her feet in 5 years!

When I applied them to her spine and asked her how she was doing she said, "Having MS is like living with a monster whispering in my ear 24/7 and at that particular moment I don't hear the monster." It was very powerful for both of us.

In addition to Raindrop I use a whole variety of oils with my clients. If someone is suffering from sciatica I use cistus and peppermint. If an athlete is aching I'll use black pepper oil, copaiba and Idaho balsam fir. For general pain I use Deep Relief and Stress Away; the relief is almost instantaneous. Those are just a few of many, many oils I use depending upon the client and their issues.

I have skied for years and my knees began to give me a lot of pain. In addition, as a massage therapist your body takes a lot of abuse and I was beginning to feel discomfort in my hips, back, wrists, etc. I had been using the oils to get relief but the pain would come back. One day a bottle of Ningxia Red (antioxidant, whole food beverage) arrived with my order because of a promotion the company was having. My husband and I began drinking one ounce per day and within two weeks my pain was completely gone.

As a parent, though, there is one instance that really stands out for me. Our family had arrived home from a vacation and my son, Kenny, was anxious to go see his friends. He hopped on his bike and took off out of the driveway at the same time our neighbor was coming down the road. Neither one of them saw each other and my son got hit by the car, flew over the windshield and onto the ground. My husband and Kenny's twin brother saw the entire thing.

They got him out of the road, onto the grass and called the ambulance. I wasn't home at the time but my husband called me while waiting for the ambulance. In that moment I remembered some information from a seminar entitled "Dr. Mom's Oils" by a Dr. Peter Minke regarding Valor oil and trauma. Specifically you should put the oil on the exact location that the trauma occurs. I told my husband to pour Valor on Kenny's legs where they were swelling. My husband told me that before his eyes the swelling went down and the bruising pulled back. When I got to the hospital and looked at Kenny's legs, there were holes the size of dimes in them yet there was no blood whatsoever. It was amazing and even the doctors and nurses in the hospital were puzzled.

That night we diffused Dream Catcher (an oil blend) when Kenny went to sleep. A couple hours later my husband and I were going up to bed ourselves and stopped in the room to check on him. He opened his eyes and said, "I just had the greatest dream. Meredith (cousin) came over to visit me and brought a movie and popcorn. When we got finished with the movie I looked down and my legs were completely healed." Of course, they weren't but what a great dream for him to have. The whole experience was one we will never forget and I firmly believe that without essential oils the outcome would not have been as good.

For over 4 years now I have incorporated Young Living Essential Oils into every area of our lives. The oils have literally become a lifestyle for us and, of course, with helping clients on a daily basis.

Victorina Bostelaar, Lake MacQuarie, NSW, Australia

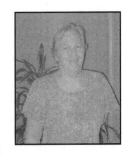

I am a registered nurse, and since the 1970's I have studied and worked with alternative healing modalities. One day a friend rang me up and said, "There's meeting about essential oils. These oils must be very good because my wife has already bought some. Are you interested in coming to a meeting?" I said, "Oh, yes, of course."

The speaker at that meeting was Alan Simpson. I was so impressed by what I heard I immediately signed up for a kit of oils. As soon as the oils arrived I bought the Essential Oil Desk Reference and began studying. I started using the oils here and there but hadn't had any particular "ah-ha" moment until a situation with my grandson arose. He was 13 at that time and accidentally hit his thumb with a hammer. He knew I had oils and asked me "Can you do something about it?" I really didn't know what would work on a banged up finger so I first tried lavender oil but it didn't make a difference. Then I tried PanAway and, again, nothing. I was beginning to feel like a failure but then remembered something that Gary Young, the founder, said in one of his lectures; "if one doesn't work, try the next and the next. There's one that will work." So I grabbed Aroma Siez, and tried that one. The second it hit his thumb, he said, "The pain is gone." He never complained anymore. So, that was my first "miracle" of the oils.

Sometime after that I made the mistake of eating a Filet O'
Fish from McDonald's. I ended up with food poisoning.
I didn't just feel bad—I was actually in pain, agony to be
exact. Two days went by and I was still lying in bed feeling
sorry for myself when it finally dawned on me, "I have
the essential oils." So I grabbed the blend called DiGize
and took several drops internally as well as rubbing some
on my stomach. Within an hour I was out of pain, up and
feeling normal. I continued with the DiGize for several
days and never had a relapse. This particular situation really
blew my mind. Now I cannot live without Young Living
Essential Oils. Even my grandchildren are now asking for
the oils or inquiring, "What do I use for this or that?" My
granddaughter recently had a baby and immediately asked
me to get her some Gentle Baby for the child. Recently I
gave all my children a diffuser and oils for Christmas. It is
the best gift you can give someone. Whatever the situation
is, there is an oil for it! A healthy, natural way to heal.

Perri Winkel, Adamstown, NSW, Australia

I had been an essential oil user for many
years when I came across Young Living.
I was trying to locate a hard to find oil,
called hyssop, which Young Living had
and I immediately bought. The reason I
wanted hyssop was because one of my
four children had a continual cough that
flared at bedtime, would wake her and

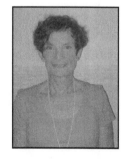

disturb her sleep. By diffusing hyssop before she went to bed it completely stopped her from coughing.

I really liked the quality of the Young Living oils and began purchasing others. My other daughter would get a cold sore about every six months and nothing we ever tried worked, as anyone who suffers from these knows. They end up sticking around for weeks. One day I decided to try geranium when she just started getting that tingling feeling at the beginning of a cold sore. It went away almost immediately. Some months later the same thing; just as the cold sore was starting we used geranium and it instantly went away. She was 9 years old when we had those two applications. She is now 25 years old and she has never gotten another cold sore in her life!

Obviously I have been using Young Living essential oils for a very long time now. I have realized that the Young Living brand is just more powerful than any other oils I previously used. It may sound extreme to someone who doesn't use them but I would not be without essential oils. I don't have to use Ibuprofen for headaches or menstrual cramps; I haven't been to the dentist in 20 years because I use essential oils on my gums and teeth, as well as the Young Living Dentarome Toothpaste. I know my health is better today because of Young Living Essential Oils.

Nicole O'Malley, Charlestown, RI, USA

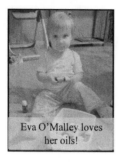

Eva O'Malley loves her oils!

We were first introduced to essential oils through friends. I was a new mother with a three month old baby. During those first three months my daughter had been admitted to the hospital where we had been given more misdiagnosis than answers. I was frustrated with the 'system,' was searching for answers and solutions, and knew I wanted better, more natural options for my family.

One of the issues we were dealing with was my daughter had been born with a severe tongue tie. This made nursing/breastfeeding very difficult for both of us. We received lactation support which helped some but did nothing for my very poor milk supply. My doctor recommended medications but I was not willing to take them; I wanted a less invasive option. Another issue was my daughter had horrible acid reflux and from one week of age she had been on Zantac, a prescription medication. I was not comfortable with this but did not know of any other options for her. She had to keep her food down in order to get nutrition.

The friends who introduced us to essential oils had a biofeedback machine that identified stressors in the body. There was nothing invasive about it so I took the opportunity to have my daughter tested on it. Although I was overwhelmed by the amount of information it gave us, it provided us with some answers and a direction to move towards. We immediately ordered the Young Living Essential 7 Kit as well as an oil blend called Di-Gize (for my daughter), fennel (for me—lactation support), wintergreen (for my husband), Kidscents body wash, and every Thieves product they sold!

We began to use the oils and soon were able to determine the best way to use the oils for each of us. We noticed some immediate changes. My daughter, who had always been extremely constipated, was able to have regular bowel movements simply by me ingesting a few drops of Di-Gize! (So, she was receiving the Di-Gize through drinking my breast milk) My very poor milk supply increased from approximately 11oz/day to around 17oz/day. My daughter eventually came off of the Zantac. My husband began using wintergreen for his chronic neck and back pain and three herniated disks and also became hooked. My daughters 'cradle cap' cleared up very quickly. I believe this happened because the change in body-wash and cleaning products in our household. We were all hooked.

Our "collection" of oils has vastly increased over the past year and a half. My now 18 month old daughter is even captivated and constantly asks for her "doop doops". (A name she associated because when I applied oils to her I would say "doop, doop" as they dropped from the bottle.) I am happy and proud to say that we no longer have any conventional medication or toxic cleaning products in our house.

Friends may chuckle at first when we offer them wintergreen or basil in place of Tylenol for a headache but it doesn't take long for them to understand why we made the switch. Other mothers are constantly asking about what I put on (both myself and my daughter) to make us smell so good. Panicked mothers who drop the ever important binky or favorite toy in the mall often leave with one of my thieves spray bottles that I keep stashed everywhere. I am excited to raise my daughter knowing that there are more natural approaches to healing and hope that she continues with her fondness for "doop doops".

Nigel Pendrigh, Penang, Malaysia

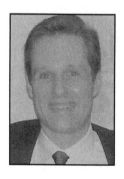

My introduction to the oils was probably like a lot of guys, through their wife. She and her friends would get together at the house with these "smelly things." I stayed as far away as possible, because it reminded of the perfume department in Macy's. But I like to think I'm not an idiot and it was impossible not to see what was happening to people when they smelled the oils and when they applied them on their body. Profound changes were visible. So I quickly realized that the oils were actually having an effect, a therapeutic effect. More and more people were benefitting from them and raving about it to their friends.

Testimonials

My first personal use of the oils came because of my love-hate relationship with mosquitoes; they love me, I hate them. Within a few hours of being bitten I will have a welt half an inch wide and a tenth of an inch high (1.5 centimeters by 1 millimeter) about the size of a US five cent piece I could somewhat control my scratching during the day but while sleeping I would scratch myself. As a result they would last for weeks before healing. Of course I had tried every cream and potion available—even things from the chemist—but nothing really helped. Then I decided to try the oils. I discovered that if I put just one drop of Young Living's lavender oil on within a half an hour or so of being bitten it would be down to the size of a pinhead within 3 hours. And there was no more itching. That really got my attention.

One of the other products that initially amazed me was the Thieves blend of oil. We live in a really humid place and when we would leave for a holiday or business travel, within two to four weeks we would come home to mold on everything—leather, plastic, clothes, you name it. It didn't matter what supermarket product we had used, even bleach, things still got moldy. We began using the Thieves Household Cleaner. We use it in the dishwasher, the clothes washer, on the floor, washing the walls, windows, cupboards—everything—even in the car. Now we come home to a clean, mold-free house. It is fantastic.

Karlie Gilbert, Jamisontown, NSW, Australia

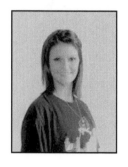

My favorite oil without a doubt would have to be PanAway. I have been dancing since I was 4 years old and around age 14 I was told I needed to have a knee operation, costing around $20,000, or I would never be able to dance again. My dream of being a dancer was crushed! My Mum was a single parent with 3 kids, so there was no way that was going to happen. As a result, I continued dancing for as long as I could and stopped at the age of 18.

By age 20 I was experiencing really chronic hip pain. I went to a physiotherapist and got x-rays. It turns out that all of my knee pain was actually due to my hips being out of alignment. So I had an explanation for the pain but no solution. I tried every pain killer available—even prescriptions—and nothing would ease the pain. I was losing sleep and being unable to do so many things. I was frustrated and decided to look at other options.

A friend of mine gave me the essential oil PanAway to try. Within 20 minutes of using this oil I felt absolutely NO pain at all. After three days of using this oil I was sleeping through the night and could begin doing things physically that I hadn't in a long time. I now have been using Young Living oils for 3 years and am now a Dance teacher and continue to dance in shows; just like I was 14 again! Young

Living oils have changed my life and have let me pursue my dream once again.

Trish Herreen, Glenelg, SA, Australia

I was introduced to Young Living Essential Oils at a time when I was fearful and frustrated that a number of long term persistent health issues were not responding to conventional or alternative treatments. I had seemingly exhausted all avenues that might turn things around. Then, a live blood 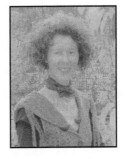 analysis revealed that I had sluggish lymphatics.

I was then introduced to Sharon Neal in Adelaide, South Australia at a demonstration of the Raindrop Technique, which involved the application of a series of specific essential oils to increase circulation, oxygenation and immunity at a cellular level. After seeing the demonstration I booked in for a Raindrop treatment. During my first massage, as the oils were applied to my feet, I became aware of activity in my brain. This lead me to a new understanding of the profound healing capacity of these oils on a physical, emotional and energetic level simultaneously.

I continued with the Raindrop Technique, started applying the oils myself, and began taking Omega Blue, Inner

Defense, Longevity, and NingXia Red supplements. Inner Defense capsules are my favorite, which contain the oils of clove, oregano, thyme, lemongrass, lemon, eucalyptus radiata, rosemary and cinnamon bark, boosting my immune system. In the six weeks that I've been using the oils and oil based supplements, my gluten intolerance has transformed from three days of bloating, dysentery, headache, increased temperature, mouth ulcers and fatigue to half a day of fatigue. My body is definitely stronger with increased immunity and continues to transform at the cause level and heal the symptoms that were previously immovable. This has provided me with a great sense of relief, restoration and gratitude to have finally found the missing link to my health, vitality and sustainable wellbeing.

Rochelle Judd, Ashfield, NSW, Australia

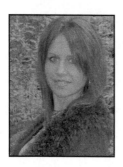

When I was introduced to Young Living Essential Oils four years ago I wasn't new to the concept of aromatherapy. Many years ago I had burned oils to make the house smell pretty or would put a few drops in a bath for relaxation. For no particular reason I lost interest.

My first few experiences with therapeutic grade essential oils quickly led me to believe these oils were more than just a pretty smell! I was unfortunate enough to be bitten by a spider on my chest. A year prior to this I had a similar bit and it took over 6 months to heal. New to the oils I did some reading and decided to use a blend of oils called Purification. I applied one or two drops of the oil, undiluted, and an hour later I couldn't even find the spot where I had been bitten! Given my previous experience I thought to myself, "This is miraculous."

My next experience with the oils related to my chronic colds and flu's; I had been getting at least 5 a year and simply suffered through because I knew how bad most of the chemist capsules are for you. Someone told me that they put 10 drops of an oil blend called Thieves in a capsule at the first signs of sickness. The next time I felt a cold coming on I did just that and "BINGO," no cold. I was truly amazed because to me it seemed like magic. And to thing that it was 100% natural was just incredible. These two experiences led me to really begin reading and learning more about therapeutic grade essential oils.

But the experience that got me to really take notice was around a migraine headache. These excruciating headaches were not new to me and I typically would take pain killers. Even though I had these other positive experiences with the oils I thought to myself, "This is too big for the oils, I need real medication!" So I decided to take 4 pain killers. Interestingly enough, this time my body repelled them, as I went straight upstairs and vomited. At that point the oils were my only option and I located a blend called MGrain. I rubbed it into both sides of my neck and shoulders and went to bed. About fifteen minutes went by and the next thing I knew it was morning. For me this was truly amazing because often these headaches would linger for several days.

Like many people I initially had been skeptical about the ability of an oil to be therapeutic. All these physical applications were a testament to their effectiveness. Then I was given a powerful emotional experience. I am typically a very happy, forgiving person but had just gone through a betrayal situation that hurt deeply. I was wallowing in my pain and unhappiness and was simply miserable and unable to let go and move on. My husband (at the time), who was highly skeptical of the oils sarcastically said to me, "haven't you got an oil for that?" I wasn't appreciative of his comment but it is what I needed at the time and I replied, "As a matter of fact I do!"

 In my kit there was an oil blend called Joy. When I first had seen it I remember thinking to myself, "Yea, right; as if an oil can actually make you happy." I opened the bottle and rubbed some on my chest and then rubbed my hands together and breathed in the aroma. Within seconds I could feel my mood lifting and felt a smile coming on. Then I actually began laughing. My husband said came into the room and asked, "Is that the oil?" "I guess so," I replied and gave him some. He didn't laugh but he did have a big, cheesy grin on his face. I don't know a lot of technical information about the oils but I do know that from that moment on, I was freed from my grudge.

Now I have too many amazing stories to tell. Probably easiest simply to say that Young Living Essential Oils have impacted and changed my life in many ways; physically, emotionally and spiritually. Even more so, I enjoy watching the oils bless so many of my friends and family by using these natural God given gifts of nature! It is truly a blessing.

Sharon Neal, Carey Gully, SA, Australia

I was first introduced to Young Living oils by a fellow practitioner, who knew I had an aroma-therapist background. We were both attending a 4-day workshop together and she began to discuss with me the purity of Young Living oils. I ended up purchasing frankincense, peppermint and lavender. 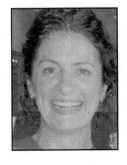 I carried them in my handbag as a first aid kit for the next several years.

Several years later I was working with another group of practitioners who gave me a much greater exposure to Young Living oils. It is at this point where I really began to appreciate the purity of Young Living oils and their vibrational healing qualities.

At this particular time I had been in and out of a toxic personal relationship for 18 months. This was causing me constant emotional, spiritual, mental and physical imbalances and was depleting my immune system. I began having extreme kidney pain, which led to two emergency visits where they tried to patch me up. Unsuccessful I ended up admitted to the hospital where they pumped me with morphine injections and intravenous antibiotics for three days.

When I was released a girlfriend collected me from the hospital and dropped me off at home. Unfortunately I returned to receive no support on any level my boyfriend. It was a nightmare of an experience.

I was in a toxic environment in every sense of the word but it still took me several months to finally build up enough courage and strength to leave the relationship and the home my partner and I were living in. I had to salvage what was left of me, my sanity and my health!

As part of my healing I was using essential oils. Most of my choices were intuitive and designed to support my severely depleted energy levels. I must admit, although I had about a dozen different Young Living oils I was still using some of the other brands of 'pure' essential oils I still owned.

I invested in the Essential Oil Desk Reference to increase my education about the oils. It was after reading through this book that I read about the Young Living Feelings Kit! (A kit of oils specifically for emotional support.) I also finally understood the importance of essential oil purity and stopped using the other brands of oils. I started using the Feelings Kit oils morning and night and soon after discovered that Young Living essential oils were my savoir during this transition. I was able to put closure on my previous relationship.

I was feeling better but knew my body was still toxic. I went on a 20-day detox and also continued my feelings essential oil ritual for the next 6-8 weeks. I eventually progressed to a daily ritual sequence of oils designed for 'letting go.' I also used other oils intuitively to support me when necessary. I followed this ritual for approximately 8-10 weeks at the same time I was also performing between 10-15 Raindrop Techniques a week on my clients. After this I undertook many EECT sessions on myself, which allowed the oils another method of releasing my emotional baggage. Yes, it was a lot but I was doing everything I possibly could to supporting detoxifying my body on all levels.

It worked! Over this period of time I gradually became clearer on all levels. I was calmer, more stable, and able to remain strong during stressful situations. In particular I was able to avoid being drawn back into the toxic personal relationship that had previously had me hooked beyond release!

My body physically regained its strength both internally and externally. I was maintaining a healthy weight and glowing complexion.

The oils have allowed me to finally connect with my authentic self and my true purpose in this lifetime. They have supported me on a physical, mental, emotional, and spiritual level allowing my body, mind, hormones, and faith to be rebuilt. I now have a strengthened foundation with which to build a powerful future of being a messenger for the gift Young Living oils purity and vibrational self-healing properties can offer humanity!

Liz Garrett, Virginia Beach, VA, USA

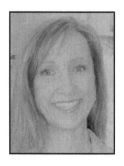

I used essential oils for decades and did not understand the difference high-quality, pure, therapeutic-grade oils could make. At a party (of all places), a friend offered Young Living Frankincense oil for my husband's ganglion cyst. At the time he had this cyst for over a year and no essential oil that I had previously tried had even the slightest effect on the cyst. To the amazement (and amusement) of everyone at the party, within hours of applying the Young Living Frankincense the cyst began shrinking noticeably

This really got my attention. Of course, my husband was thrilled to be rid of the cyst.

I started replacing my old oils with Young Living oils and, for the first time, started experiencing real relief for insomnia, headaches, indigestion, sore muscles, etc. I confess I can be thick-headed. No amount of talking or reading could have convinced me the way these results did. Pure, therapeutic-grade essential oils work. Period.

Kimberly Seeto, Croydon, NSW, Australia

I am a Massage Therapist and a big believer in natural health and healing. I knew essential oils played an important role in accelerated healing and wanted to begin incorporating essential oils into my massage treatments. After coming across Young Living essential oils at a Health Care Expo, I have never looked back.

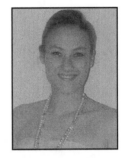

My first experience with the essential oils was with Deep Relief. I was driving one Sunday on the way to my soccer game when I felt a sudden onset of sharp pain in my knee. I tried rubbing the area with my hand but the pain wasn't subsiding. As a midfielder in my soccer team I do a lot of running and I started to worry that I wasn't going to be able to play. I didn't want to let my team mates down. I remembered that I had just received a Deep Relief roll-on in my kit and happened to have it in my bag. Within a few seconds of applying the oil my pain had dissipated. I wondered how long before the pain returned, but I was able to play a full game of soccer pain free. I really couldn't believe how quickly it had worked, and the smell is amazing. This is where I started to fall in love with Young

Living Essential Oils. Now I carry Deep Relief everywhere I go.

My next amazing experience with the oils was when my mum (58), injured her back at work. She works with children so it's important for her to be able to bend down and move around to interact with the children. One day she picked up one of the kids to do a nappy (diaper) change and felt a sharp pain shoot straight across her lower back. As the day went on, the pain became worse and unbearable, bringing her to tears. I picked her up from work early because she was in no state to drive. She was in agonising pain and could hardly move. Sitting down and standing up became a struggle and she could hardly bend forwards to reach for her toes. She said she felt like a 90-year old woman!

I took her to the doctors and they told her it was just muscular. They gave her a prescription for anti-inflammatories and a referral to the physio. She was told to stay out of work for a week and rest. When we got home we put an ice pack on her back and I suggested to her that before she takes all these medications we try the oils first and see what happens. I didn't have many oils at the time but felt that clove, peppermint and wintergreen would be sensible choices. After just one day of using these oils her pain had eased considerably but was not completely gone. After the second day the pain had almost disappeared. She was able to move more freely and could bend forward reaching to her knees without discomfort. She was also able to finally sleep. After the third day the pain had completely gone and mum was almost back to normal range of movement. She was back to herself again pain free. I was amazed and shocked at how fast her recovery was! Mum couldn't believe it either. By using essential oils she didn't need to take any pharmaceutical medications or go to a physio. Best of all she was back to work after just three days.

I believe I was guided to Young Living essential oils that day at the Health Care Expo in Sydney. Since then I use oils every day and gain a greater appreciation for their power and the impact they have on your health. Working with them has been life-changing. Now I avoid synthetic products as much as I can, knowing that my body is much better off and healthier with natural, essential oil products instead. And even knowing how great they are, I still get amazed every time I see how wonderfully they work. Thank you Gary Young and Young Living Essential Oils.

Lisa Taylor, Cushing, MN, USA

I was introduced to Young Living Essential oils when a friend of mine invited me to attend a class on Everyday Oils. The person speaking started talking about using lavender oil for allergies. I suffered from severe allergies. Every Spring I would basically have to stay in the house for

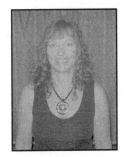

three months. I'd wake up in the morning with my eyes crusted shut. I am very sensitive to medications but my allergies were so bad that I had to take them just to get through the worst times. One time my mother gave me Claritin to try and I couldn't sleep the entire night. It was even affecting my marriage because all spring I would want the windows and doors shut and my husband would want them open; it was really hard on our relationship.

So, when I heard this Young Living distributor talk about how oils could help allergies I thought, "I'm going to get this kit of oils and take them home." I began by putting lavender on my feet and chest. I then learned about an oil blend called RC. When my allergies got bad I would put RC on my chest. That started the whole process and my symptoms began to get better. But my success was not instantaneous. I kept up with the oils but then I learned about cleansing and enzymes. I did the 5-Day Nutritive Cleanse three times in one year. I have since done the Cleansing Trio a couple of times as well. I am also using the Young Living enzymes daily. What I have noticed was that by the third spring after beginning to use Young Living products I had no allergies at all! I will sneeze for a couple of weeks but I don't have any symptoms whatsoever. I don't even use lavender anymore; I simply have no allergies.

Of course, I use oils every day and have removed as many chemicals from our lives as possible. What is interesting is that now, when I walk into a Wal-Mart or other store that have a lot of household cleaners, I not only smell them but they bother me. It's almost as if I can feel the chemicals.

Another interesting thing happened shortly after we began using the Young Living products. I noticed that a mole I had was bleeding and scabbing. I tried to get into a dermatologist, and the first available appointment was three months out. So I got hold of my up line and asked "What can I do for this?" They told me to use thyme oil topically on the mole. I had done this right before getting into the shower and quickly realized that hot, steamy water accelerates the penetration of an oil, so it burned like crazy. After that I only used lavender on it and within a month the mole was completely gone. I actually canceled my appointment! These are just two of the many benefits I have experienced using Young Living's therapeutic grade essential oils. Young Living has helped our entire family; it has truly changed our lives.

Olaf von Sperl, Castlegrag, NSW, Australia

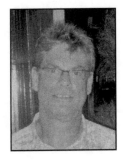

My wife had been using essential oils for years but one day she came home with a packet of the most beautiful-smelling oils. She diffused them throughout the house and used them for six or seven years before I even gave it much attention because I was skeptical as probably most males are.

Then, two years ago I went to the doctor and had a blood test. I found that I had very high cholesterol and he wanted to put me on medication. Our family doesn't like taking drugs so I went to see our naturopath. He said, "That's rubbish; start out with taking a magnesium supplement." I went home and told my wife what the naturopath had said and she in turn gave me a bunch of Young Living products to take instead of the magnesium. Of course, as a good husband you do what your wife tells you to do! The products included Omega Blue fish oil, Sulfurzyme, Ningxia Red, and lemongrass.

I followed this for over two years. Not only did I begin to feel more energized very quickly but when I finally went back to my doctor 2+ years later all my cholesterol levels had gone down to within a normal range. And the only thing I changed was using the Young Living products. I didn't even change my diet at all.

Now comes the really interesting part. When I was 18 I had a very bad sports injury that required three operations. The doctors told me I probably wouldn't ever walk properly again. I had to stop all sports and they told me to expect a knee replacement by the time I was 40. I did continue to do exercise within my limits but had always had pain that I just learned to live with. About a year into using the Young Living products I realized that the pain in my knee was gone! I can now bend my knee 90 degrees and I don't wake up anymore with a locked knee. Literally to me it feels like a new knee. I think I'll be able to do sport again.

Another personal situation involved a time when high work stress resulted in my not being able to sleep. I finally went to the doctor. He said my health was fine but he gave me a prescription for Valium as a sleep aid and added three refills. My wife, Louise, said "Rubbish" and threw it in the garbage bin. Instead she gave me a combination of valerian, lavender and RutaVala essential oils. I would rub the lavender and RutaVala under my nose and put the valerian under my tongue. Within one week I was sleeping through the night again. So, instead of having three courses of Valium, it was fixed with a few drops of essential oils.

Rebecca Bonanno, Theresa Park, NSW, Australia

I have suffered from endometriosis for years to the point where I was taking a whole week off work every month. The pain was so bad it felt like labor pains! In November of 2010 I finally got surgery but my doctor told me it would return within a year. Sadly, it was back in 8 months.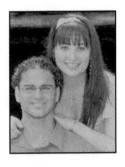

I was back to being in pain for a week every month. I was sick of taking pain killers. Sometimes I would take up to 12 Advil in one day, at least three days a month. Someone introduced me to Young Living Essential Oils and I heard on one lecture by Gary Young that Balsam Fir oil reduced inflammation. I began applying the oil every night. The next month I did not experience any pain during my menstrual cycle. I continue this routine to this day and although I sometimes have minor, "normal" menstrual pain it is not debilitating. I could not live without Young Living's Balsam Fir essential oil. It has changed my life.

Another time I had cut my hand on a piece of glass. It went in about 6mm deep and it was about 6mm wide. I applied pressure with a towel but the bleeding wouldn't stop. It was so bad that it made a pool in the palm of my hand.

The first oil I thought of was geranium. I put a drop on the cut and I could see the blood begin to clot instantly. When I rinsed my hand with water, the bleeding had completely stopped.

To ease the pain I used melaleuca alternifolia (Tea Tree) and lavender. My hand was healed within 2 days. Thank you Young Living. Three amazing oils I can't live without.

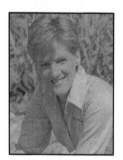 **Casey Conrad** has been in the health and fitness industry for over 25 years. She is the creator of the Take It Off Weight Loss Program, which is found in health and wellness facilities throughout North America. She is author of several books, including Winning the Struggle to Be Thin.

She has been a featured presenter in 19 countries, and is a frequent columnist for numerous industry magazines and publications.

She received her BA from The American University, her JD at Roger Williams University School of Law. In addition, she is certified in Neuro Linguistic Programming and Neuro Associative Conditioning. Casey is committed to bringing health and wellness education to individuals around the world.

Casey can be reached at YoungLivingCasey@gmail.com

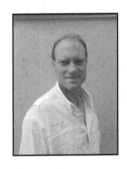

Alan Simpson has been in the health and wellness industry for 25 years. His path to the industry was far from conventional. Trained as a commercial pilot and flying instructor, a Series of health challenges led him to the study of natural healing.

For over 12 years he has been studying the science and chemistry of essential oils and has completed extensive training in Darkfield Microscopy and human cells. He has owned and operated a skin cancer research company and is currently studying as a naturopath and certified clinical aromatherapist.

Alan now travels extensively around the world, with his wife Linda; lecturing on the dangers of chemicals in our lives and on ways we can enhance our body's healing abilities. His simple, understandable approach to teaching basic quantum physics by using music as a teaching tool has earned him praise with audiences and peers alike.

Alan can be reached at YoungLivingAlan@gmail.com.